All
About
Hair

All
About
Hair

AVOIDING THE RIP-OFFS

MAKING IT BETTER

REPLACING IT IF IT'S GONE

Herbert S Feinberg, M.D.

wp

Wallingford Press

Alpine, New Jersey

For information write the publisher:
  Wallingford Press, Alpine, N.J. 07620

Photo credits: Figs. 1, 2, 25-41, author
               Figs. 14-24, Richard Pilling

Line drawings: Figs. 3-13, Spectragraphics

Produced and designed by Bernard Schleifer

Library of Congress Cataloging in Publication Data

Feinberg, Herbert S
  All about hair.

    1. Hair—Care and hygiene. 2. Baldness.
    3. Hair—Transplantation. I. Title.

RL91.F44   616.5'46   77-92355
ISBN 0-930988-01-9
0 9 8 7 6 5 4 3 2

Manufactured in the United States of America

*To my wife, Deanna,
whose help in preparing
this manuscript kept me
from tearing out my hair.*

Acknowledgments

THERE ARE MANY people who contribute in many ways to the pleasant—but often tedious—task of preparing a manuscript.

—My faithful and competent medical assistants, Mss. Laurie Cannon and Barbara Matura, R.N.

—My good friends Bob Di Iorio and Mel Gerstein, who helped with many of the "logistic" problems.

—My good friends Joe Dello Russo, M.D. and fellow hair transplanter, Ron Sherman, M.D., for their review of the many drafts.

—And finally, Ms. Gypsy da Silva for her encouragement and technical assistance in preparing the final manuscript.

Contents

REPLACING IT IF IT'S GONE

Introduction

> "If I be shaved, then my strength will leave me,
> and I shall become weak, and be like any other man."
>
> JUDGES 16

SAMSON MAY HAVE BEEN the first to worry about it. Since then, our concern about scalp hair has continued to intensify. For thousands of years, we have given our blood, purged our bowels, suffered through dietary manipulations and uncountable local remedies in an attempt to make our hair look better or avoid the kind of shedding not maliciously induced by the likes of a Delilah.

Today, in some respects, we are worse off than we were two thousand years ago when Galen suggested that we might prevent baldness by avoiding mushrooms and toadstools in our diets. We are constantly being bombarded by baldness "cures" that, along with the morass of popular misinformation about hair care, have completely confused most people who find that their hair isn't quite what they want it to be.

Avoiding the rip-offs has become increasingly difficult for the average person, who, concerned about his or her hair, has had no reliable source of information about what really can—or cannot—be done to make hair better or to grow more of it. Unfortunately, even physicians are often remiss in dispensing the sort of advice their patients deserve. This may partially explain why quackery has become so successful—estimates of the money we *waste* in seeking hair and scalp treatments run into the millions of dollars.

In order to help you solve your problems, I must first destroy the myths so effectively used by the charlatans who have confused us with their pills, diets, salves and other "restorative treatments." Once you can see through the nonsense, you'll avoid making the mistakes that seem to plague anyone who is trying to improve his or her hair or gain more of it.

Making it better requires that you understand some basic truths about why hair looks and acts the way it does, and why it may fall out. I'll also describe the various cleansing, conditioning, coloring and styling options available today, as well as many of the reliable products you can purchase to enhance the quality of your hair.

Replacing it if it's gone concerns millions of people in this country who have lost their hair. If you're looking for a way to temporarily or permanently correct your baldness, the respective sections on cosmetic and surgical hair replacement should help you.

If I can dissuade you from wasting your money on any product that promises hair growth, or if I can enlighten you about one proper styling or restorative method, you should make your investment in this book and the time spent reading it pay off many times over.

AVOIDING THE RIP-OFFS

I

Quackery

A MAGAZINE AD PROCLAIMS that there really is a way to grow hair: "I've done it and so can you." A special "nutrient" capsule, handsomely packaged is backed by numerous personal testimonials and *guaranteed* to work or triple your money back!

"A medical formula, *devised by a physician,* has reversed the chemical chain of events that causes a scalp follicle to stop producing its hair." Reported in various *newspapers* and acclaimed by other *physicians!*

"A remarkable concoction—used by *movie stars*—actually grew hair on a bald scalp." *Proof* demonstrated by before-and-after photographs!

"A series of scalp treatments advertised by clinics *specializing* in baldness." Thousands of people waste hundreds of thousands of dollars each year for the treatment of hair and scalp conditions that are either impossible to control or are easily self-treated.

All of these examples are based upon real situations. If any one of them actually delivered what they promised, this discussion would be superfluous. Each represents one of the four types of commonly practiced quackery. Amazingly, they have all been successful—in making money for the people hawking them. They, additionally, share two other characteristics—they peddle hope, and they fail to grow hair!

Understanding why these schemes succeed in fooling people should enable you to see through any other kind of nonsense therapy promoted for hair restoration. There are four rules for a successful medical flimflam. Most advertised hair-restoration schemes you encounter will be true to one or all of them.

Rule 1: The Deceptions Deal With Problems That Concern Many People.

Since baldness or "problem" hair concerns millions of people, the quacks are assured of a large consumer market.

Rule 2: The Solutions Always Appear Believable.

This is especially true for dietary schemes. Since eating vitamins, minerals, proteins and other foodstuffs is recommended as "therapy" for just about everything that ails us, why not for hair problems?

Rule 3: Scientific Facts Are Offered to Lend an Air of Credibility to It All – Cause and Effect Is Unimportant.

Since we're overburdened with facts concerning hair growth and baldness, it's easy enough to find a few to strengthen any sales pitch.

For example, the vitamin or diet "expert" will explain, quite truthfully, that vitamin E deficiency produces baldness in mice, that zinc is found in growing hair or that protein makes up the basic structure of the hair shaft. He will then assert that since *his* product contains one or more of those substances, *your* hair will regrow if it's gone or grow stronger if it's still there. Because no cause-and-effect relationship exists, his "claims" are simply never justified by the "evidence" he provides.

Rule 4: Spread the Word.

Since there is always an ample supply of gullible people around, they can do the job by word of mouth. For a more sophisticated approach, "Madison Avenue" can sell anything that's packaged properly.

The quack schemes appear faster than anyone can write about them. But as you'll find out, they all fit into one of four categories:
1. "RESTORERS" TAKEN ORALLY.
2. "RESTORERS" APPLIED DIRECTLY TO SCALP AND HAIR.
3. PHYSICAL METHODS FOR ENRICHING AND RESTORING SCALP HAIR.
4. "CLINICS" SPECIALIZING IN HAIR RESTORATION.

1

"Restorers" Taken Orally

OR, EATING YOUR WAY TO A HAIRIER SCALP

GIVEN VITAMINS, minerals or anything else that can legally be put into a capsule and sold without a prescription, someone, somewhere, will claim some sort of therapeutic benefit for it. As for dietary manipulations, the food faddists have always been able to think up ways for us to eat our way to better health and beauty. It has been estimated that we spend nearly *one-half billion* dollars a year for spurious health foods.

Hair consists essentially of protein. In addition, many minerals are present—mostly calcium, magnesium, potassium and sodium. There are also smaller quantities of cadmium, cobalt, copper, iron, lead, manganese and zinc. In addition, other substances, including vitamins, contribute to the metabolism of the hair follicle as they do for other bodily organs.

The fallacy common to the approach of eating your way to a hairier scalp is simply this: *just because a substance is required for normal growth, it does not follow that more of it will improve our well-being.*

What About Vitamin E?

Vitamin E may be the all-time winner in the "promise-everything-do-nothing" category. It has been promoted as a preventive for heart disease, a stimulant of fertility and athletic prowess, a skin healer and hair restorer.

What we *really* know about this vitamin is that its deficiency may promote anemia in small premature infants and create hair loss in *rats*.

Vitamin E is present in so many foods that no adult deficiency state has ever been described. It is estimated that if vitamin E were withheld from an adult who had been eating properly, it would take *four years* to deplete the vitamin already stored in his or her fat tissue.

Word-of-mouth and advertised therapeutic claims have increased vitamin E sales over the past few years by tens of millions of dollars. While many physicians have "suggested" that it benefits certain medical problems, it has really only proven effective for treating the anemia that may occur in premature infants. As far as stimulating hair growth in humans, it simply has never helped.

Haven't Biotin and Inositol Been Shown to Affect Hair Growth?

They are the two vitamins presently enjoying popularity as hair restorers. Like vitamin E, their deficiency has produced hair loss in *rats* and *mice*.

But like vitamin E, they are so widely available in nature that no human deficiency state has ever been described. Moreover, be wary of substances promoted for their hair-growth potential in laboratory animals. Since we are not rodents, their feeding requirements cannot readily be interpreted as being meaningful to us.

Hasn't Vitamin A Restored Scalp Hair in Humans?

Yes, if the baldness was caused by vitamin A deficiency—*or excess*. Too little or too much of this vitamin may promote poor quality scalp hair that breaks easily. Anyone suffering from a vitamin A problem, however, will usually have many other serious symptoms.

Because of its *assumed* hair growing potential and other skin benefits, vitamin A overdosage has become a vexing medical problem. So many people have poisoned themselves that the Food and Drug Administration has lowered the dosage that can be sold without a prescription.

Don't Many Physicians Prescribe Iron for Hair Loss?

Iron deficiency anemia, when *severe*, may be associated with thinning of scalp hair. Since many women who complain about thinned hair are often *slightly* iron deficient, this mineral has received wide usage by physicians. But, unfortunately, iron does not usually help. There are no reliable studies suggesting that a true correlation exists between iron deficiency and hair loss in a *normal* individual.

Isn't Zinc Quite Safe to Take?

Yes, but there's a general rule in medicine, that the "safer" a medication is the less likely it is to do anything. Zinc, however, is now being studied for the treatment of certain skin problems, including acne. While its deficiency may aggravate a type of thinning unrelated to common baldness, its role is still questionable and its therapeutic use still remains investigational. In general, for the hair problems that concern most people, all that can be truly claimed at this time is that zinc is safe, available, easy to take *and ineffective*.

What About Claims Made for Other Vitamins and Minerals Commonly Found in "Hair Restorative" Pills?

NIACIN is said to increase blood circulation in the scalp. It might—in very *high* dosages—but this still would not enhance hair growth in any significant manner.

IODINE is incorporated into many of these pills because its deficiency affects thyroid gland function, which in turn can cause hair loss. True—but if you have an iodine deficiency, you'll probably develop a goiter before you lose any hair.

FOLIC ACID and VITAMIN B 12 *deficiencies* are often claimed to affect hair growth adversely. Actually, human skin and hair are fairly insensitive to deficiencies of these vitamins.

PANTOTHENIC ACID (VITAMINS B 3 AND B 5) are supposed to help you keep your hair and its color. True—but only if you're a mouse.

Whatever hair restorative claim is made for a vitamin or mineral, chances are it's either meaningless for humans in general or anyone's specific hair problem in particular.

Hasn't Protein Deficiency Been Shown to Produce Shedding of Scalp Hair?

Yes, with the severe protein deprivation found in many underdeveloped countries, thinning of scalp hair is associated with other symptoms of malnutrition.

It's ironic that a similar kind of shedding has been reported in our well-fed society. Crash dieters subsisting on 500 to 1,000 calories a day for many weeks may experience a temporary thinning of hair. It has been suggested that their shedding is caused not by reduced calories but by inadequate protein intake. If you crash diet, don't sacrifice your dietary protein or you may sacrifice some of your hair as well.

*How About High Protein or Other Special Diets—Can They
Help to Grow Hair or Make It Stronger?*

We normally possess between 100,000 and 150,000 hairs on
our heads. For each strand, someone has either written a book
or magazine article claiming some sort of diet that can embel-
lish either the quality or quantity of our scalp hair:

- Milk, eggs and cheese top the list since they, like hair,
  consist mostly of protein.
- Vegetable oils are frequently advocated as benefactors of a
  proper coating for the hair shaft.
- Green leafy vegetables and apricots are *mandatory* if your
  hair is dry and brittle.
- And so forth.

While I imagine that eating one's way out of problem hair
can be fun, it's simply wishful thinking to count on a specific
food to strengthen your hair—unless you are severely deficient
in something that is so chemically unique that it can't be
replaced.

It is this sort of foolishness that has taken gelatin out of the
refrigerator and put it into "nail-strengthening capsules." Our
digestive systems, unfortunately, just can't utilize foodstuffs
with the specificity demanded by diet "experts."

Even if a deficiency in any vitamin, mineral or other edible
substance happens to produce shedding, the hair is always lost
throughout the *entire* scalp, and this kind of thinning is *not*
common baldness—the condition that the "hair experts" *imply*
they can help.

The miracles seem to work only for them. They all arro-
gantly assure us that only *they,* through *their* own initiative and
persistence, have discovered what scientists have not been
able to do—provide a safe oral therapy for baldness.

The only consistencies I have ever discovered in their
approach to this problem is that their "revelations," provided in
a pill or book, will cost you money and make them wealthy.

2

"Restorers" Applied Directly to Scalp and Hair

OR, FEEDING YOUR FOLLICLES

SKIN, AND ITS TWO offshoots—hair and nails—being completely visible and accessible, is well suited for treatments applied directly to it. The medical profession and the cosmetic industry, recognizing this fact, have created many excellent topical preparations for various skin, hair and nail diseases or cosmetic problems.

The charlatans, however, have also appreciated the ease with which hair and scalp can be anointed. Realizing that people love to medicate themselves, they have created scores of hair "restorers" with which they've swindled the public out of millions of dollars.

The fallacy common to their approach is that hair or its follicles can be "fed" by rubbing something into the scalp. Enough enzymes, vitamins, protein, carbohydrate and even manure have been applied to people's scalps to fertilize the Sahara desert. But, as you will soon realize, you can't "feed" your follicles. It really doesn't work—except in only one special circumstance that I'll discuss below.

Doesn't It Seem Logical to Treat the Scalp Directly When Its Hairs Aren't Growing Properly?

Yes, it does. But our skin, in order to keep us secure from our environment, provides a formidable barrier to the penetration of anything rubbed into it. For a substance to reach the depth of the hair follicle, it must be prepared in concentrations that are very high or put into special solutions that can easily pass through the skin barrier. Nothing sold over the counter, despite claims to the contrary, has ever been shown to do this effectively.

Why The Special Interest in Hormones to Reverse the Balding Tendency?

Another name for common baldness is "male-pattern" baldness. The term "male" refers to male hormone. Without its presence, the tendency for someone to bald will not be realized.

This fact provides us with a simple but devastating solution for the problem of baldness in men—castration! Deprived of his male organs, a castrated man (eunuch) may find solace only in the possession of a hairy scalp. His scalp hair, however, must be present *before* castration, because this operation will *not* grow hair on a bald scalp.

Several decades ago, in certain mid-western states, men having certain types of mental illness could legally be castrated if they were institutionalized. A group of these eunuchs, varying widely in age and density of scalp hair, were studied.

A man destined to bald, who was castrated in his early twenties while he still had most of his hair, lost very little hair as he aged. If, at age forty, he was given male hormone, he shed all the hair he *was supposed to have lost* over that twenty-year period but within several months.

Other eunuchs, matched for age and hair distribution, but without this tendency for baldness, lost little or no hair when given male hormone. How this hormone acts on susceptible hair follicles to allow them to bald, was not understood then. It is still unclear today.

Does This Mean That Bald Men Are Actually More Masculine?

Unfortunately, it doesn't follow that "bald is better." While the sex hormones do influence the growth and density of scalp and body hair, the key factor concerns the kind of hair follicles you possess. For example, orientals grow less body hair than caucasians, but this reflects the status of their hair follicles, not their male hormone production.

While a balding man cannot lose his hair without his male hormones, he cannot assume that these hormones are circulating at *super* levels. Conversely, a man with a full head of hair needn't feel guilty. His follicles are simply strong enough to withstand the effects of *any* concentration of male hormone.

But, Women Go Bald. Do They Have Male Hormones?

Yes, they have. *All women produce male-type hormones in their ovaries and adrenal glands* in amounts reaching about 25% of the levels found in men. Since their higher levels of female hormones (estrogens) somehow cancel out the balding effects of male hormone, most women escape the problem, which is certainly more common in men.

If, however, a young woman has a strong tendency for baldness, her *normally low levels* of male hormone may affect her scalp follicles adversely. As women age, their female hormone levels drop, offering less protection against their unchanging levels of male hormone. Accordingly, the incidence of common baldness increases for women around the menopause. Many women, middle-aged and older, develop common baldness in a very characteristic pattern. As you'll see later, the pattern is different from that seen in a man, but it is the same condition influenced by the same factor—male hormone.

Aren't Many Physicians Injecting Female Hormone into People's Scalps to Slow Down Hair Loss?

Over the past few years, physicians specializing in baldness have injected various kinds of female hormones, in *very dilute concentrations*, directly into the scalp in an attempt to block the action of male hormone upon the hair follicle.

Many people receiving these "hormone shots" are convinced that they've impeded their hair loss. I, like many other physicians, have had patients who thought that they shed less hair or grew more hair during prolonged therapy. There is, however, *no objective evidence* that this is so. Any success has probably been more coincidental than real—especially when we remember that the *normal fluctuation* of daily hair fall may vary between just a few and up to fifty or sixty hairs a day.

Isn't There Any Way That Female Hormone Might Work Applied Directly to the Scalp?

This is the "special circumstance" mentioned above.

If *high dosages* of female hormone are either injected or, as a lotion, rubbed directly into a man's scalp, the shedding associated with common baldness might stop.

But this approach creates a serious problem. Because so much hormone must be used, it would be absorbed into his body. In other words, it would act as if it were being given orally. The man might grow vigorous hair, but his "vigor" would end there—for he would become a "chemical castrate" and suffer side effects which include loss of libido and signs of feminization such as breast enlargement and changes in the male pattern of body hair distribution.

How About Using Concentrated Hormone Lotions for Women?

It would appear that women should fare better with this type of approach. The problem again focuses upon absorption of estrogen into the body.

Since we're really asking, "Does this hormone help when given orally?" the answer is, "It might help, but the high dosages and the many years required to take estrogens would probably create undesirable side effects such as blood clots and a higher risk of female-organ cancer." Besides, when used in the "safe" dosage range, I have never seen a healthy young or menopausal woman, losing her hair from common baldness, actually helped by estrogens.

But Don't Many Pregnant Women or Women Taking Birth Control Pills Lose Less Hair?

They often do. The reason is that during pregnancy, or the "pseudo-pregnancy" induced by birth control pills, hair, now influenced by higher levels of estrogens, will have a tendency to grow for longer periods of time so that fewer "resting hairs" will be found on the scalp. A single hair grows for about three years, rests for three months, then falls out. Fewer resting hairs mean fewer falling hairs.

It is the sudden decrease in the level of female hormone that accounts for the hair fall following pregnancy or discontinuation of birth control pills. At this time, all the hairs that should have entered their resting stage earlier do so all at once and shedding occurs.

Luckily, young women—the ones most likely to become pregnant or be taking birth control pills—rarely suffer from common baldness. If they have this tendency, the birth control pill might help for a while, but eventually the hairs would have to stop growing and begin to fall out again.

Recently, a new type of oral contraceptive, the "mini-dose" pill, containing chemicals more like male-type hormone rather than estrogen, has been introduced. A woman having a strong family background of common baldness might now lose her hair like her father while on this pill. Consult your gynecologist!

Several Years Ago, Some Physicians Reported New Hair Growth After Male Hormone Had Been Rubbed into Scalps.

Interesting—and true. Physicians may not always be guiltless of contributing to the general confusion about hair growth.

What actually occurred was that a few hair follicles *that still had the potential to grow one more cycle of hair* were somehow induced to thrive one last time. At best, a bald scalp might produce about ten or twenty such hairs—not nearly enough to create the kind of excitement that this report generated.

The publicity was unfortunate, because many people were misled into trying something that just didn't work.

Don't Many Physicians Prescribe Other Types of Lotions for Hair Loss?

Disregarding the lotions used for treatment of skin conditions often associated with hair loss, such as psoriasis, there are two kinds of medical approaches that require comment.

The first is the "try this" approach offered by the well-meaning doctor faced with an apprehensive patient losing his or her hair. The doctor, feeling sorry for his patient, often attempts to soften the "shock" of discovering that baldness has begun by prescribing some sort of bland therapy. This may consist of supplemental iron, ultraviolet light treatments to the scalp or one of many innocuous lotions rubbed onto one's head. There is really no substitute for firm explanations and sympathetic reassurance when dealing with this problem.

The other "medical" approach is offered by physicians—and their number, luckily, is very few—who are no better than the rest of the quacks promising to restore hair. They usually have "discovered" something such as a hormone, vitamin, etc., that may even require a prescription. Their formulas are quite secret, and the results of their startling discoveries have never been published in a medical journal or verified in a proper scientific study.

If you hear about a physician—or for that matter anyone or any product—purporting to restore your lost hair, call your local county medical society. They may be able to advise you directly, check it out for you or refer you to a competent physician specializing in hair problems.

Isn't There Any Hope of Discovering a Baldness Cure That Can Be Put Into a Lotion to Be Applied Directly to the Scalp?

Yes, there are studies being performed today to search for a safe, effective way to reverse the balding tendency without resorting to medication taken internally.

Since we know that male hormone is necessary for baldness to develop, researchers are trying to find a substance that will have "anti-male hormone" effects when applied to the scalp without interfering with other bodily functions.

One such group of anti-male hormones is already being studied for the treatment of prostate cancer. Since men with this disease do better when given female hormone, other drugs have been developed that suppress male hormone without the feminizing effects of estrogens. Most of these "anti-hormones" have other toxic side effects that so far have precluded their use for a cosmetic problem such as baldness. But hopefully, the chemists will eventually produce the ultimate drug that will do the job safely.

This kind of anti-male hormone research is exciting and encouraging. We're now starting to ask the right questions, and some of the early answers appear promising. But the anti-baldness product you'll be able to buy in your local drug store *hasn't been discovered yet.* Furthermore, this discovery will probably be made by bona fide scientists, reporting their findings in medical journals, rather than "bath tub chemists" conjuring up "hair restorers" that will be advertised in your local newspapers.

3

Physical Methods For Enriching and Restoring Scalp Hair

OR, MASSAGING YOUR WAY TO A HAIRIER SCALP

"A HUNDRED STROKES a day!"

This old dictum directed the grooming habits of many young girls who were admonished to brush their hair in this manner in order to "strengthen" it and make it "shine." This concept of brushing your hair or massaging your scalp to enhance growth or attractiveness is still with us today. It's based on a popular misconception that scalp stimulation will increase blood flow to make hair grow faster and stronger and will increase oil gland activity to lubricate hair more effectively.

But Isn't Baldness Associated With a Decreased Blood Supply to the Scalp?

Yes. The older we get and the balder we become, the fewer blood vessels remain in the scalp. But just because a diminished blood supply is associated with baldness, it doesn't necessarily follow that one causes the other. In fact, the scalp, bald or hairy, still receives more blood than it needs. The success of hair transplants has proven that the baldest scalp can easily nurture growing follicles when they are moved into it.

Doesn't Hair Grow Faster and to Greater Lengths if the Blood Supply to Its Skin Is Increased?

Yes, this may occur in children who, congenitally, have greater numbers of blood vessels in an arm or leg. The affected limb grows larger than its mate and its hairy cover may become quite exuberant.

Can't Scalp Massage Stimulate Hair Growth in the Same Way?

A youthful bald scalp is not really "bald." It is covered by the same short hairs that make up the "peach fuzz" covering our foreheads. These baby-fine soft hairs are the products of very small hair follicles quite unlike the giants that produce our normal scalp hairs that are capable of growing for up to eight years to lengths of several feet.

The "fuzz" follicles have very short growth cycles yielding hairs that grow only to about $1/16$ inch. When stimulated by frequent massaging, they may lengthen, reaching perhaps ¼ inch and no more.

Any physical method that promises to grow hair on a bald scalp may work, but quadrupling the length of a $1/16$ inch hair, and perhaps thickening it a bit, is not exactly what people are hoping to accomplish.

I remember one highly touted product that was written about in a national magazine, endorsed by movie stars and accompanied by photographs demonstrating "remarkable hair growth." The "miracle" was provided by a close-up lens that enlarged the ¼-inch hairs to change their actual perspective in relation to the scalp. The pictures of the magnified hairs looked impressive, but they could never be useful as a scalp cover.

What Kind of Products Are Associated With This Method?

I classify these as the "time-and-money wasters."

The mechanical gimmicks usually include vibrators and special brushes that are used in a "massage program."

They may be sold with or without "restorative" hair products, usually made up as shampoos or lotions. These latter products are as useless as any other "hair restorer" you can buy over the counter. They serve only as vehicles for the massage program, incidentally increasing profits since they are used up and replaced during the treatment time, usually extending for months.

Can Brushing or Massaging the Scalp Stimulate Oil Gland Activity, Adding Luster to the Hair?

Very slightly. While a minimal amount of brushing might distribute the oil present on hairs more evenly, the scalp's oil glands cannot be "milked." They secrete slowly and at a fairly constant rate. If your scalp and hair are too dry, there are simpler and safer ways to compensate for the lack of natural oils (see SECTION III).

Can Frequent Brushing or Massaging Be Harmful?

Both kinds of physical manipulations may produce results that are opposite to what you expect.

Vigorous, short-term massaging, brushing or back-combing (teasing) may shear the hair shafts, creating a diffuse hair loss.

Less vigorous, long-term manipulations are often associated with protracted tension that tends to disturb the sensitive growing scalp follicles. Many of them may enter their resting stage prematurely, resulting in more falling hairs. *Increased* shedding is not exactly what anyone hopes to achieve by massaging and brushing.

4

"Clinics" Specializing in Hair Restoration

OR, SCALPING YOUR POCKETBOOK

WE JOKE ABOUT THE bald barber telling us how to grow hair. But what if he weren't bald. Would his opinions be taken more seriously? Surrounded by the tonsorial tools and furnishings of his trade, a barber or hairdresser could pass himself off as a specialist in hair restoration. Luckily, these people, being sensible and honest, usually concentrate on cutting hair rather than saving it.

The operators of hair clinics, however, take full advantage of our tendencies to look for "experts" to solve our problems.

The word "clinic" implies therapy. Modified by such terms as "hair restoration" or "hair specialists," the added implication becomes that of expertise and hope.

The clinic establishments are almost always set up with the kind of furnishings and equipment that suggest professionalism.

The advertising that baits the customer is usually both clever and deceptive.

To enhance their personal image, the individuals running these clinics may call themselves "trichologists" *(tri-koló-jist,* one who studies hair). Physicians specializing in hair disorders never refer to themselves by this officious title, nor can a university bestow it upon anyone. The term is usually embraced by the self-styled "experts," who exaggerate their professional qualifications in a way that never approaches the knowledge they actually possess.

Over the years, many hair clinics, aided by deceitful advertising, have become the prime purveyors of hair and scalp quackery. Millions of dollars are spent yearly in these establishments, yet the problems people bring there could be handled for a fraction of this cost. If everyone understood how little they actually accomplish, these clinics would rarely find a customer.

What Services Do These Clinics Offer?

They usually claim that they can control or prevent baldness.

They may also "treat" various scalp conditions, such as dandruff, oily hair and itching.

Unfortunately, they usually deal with these problems by offering many of the "nonsense therapies" I've discussed in the first three chapters.

Recently, some of them have extended their services to include hair weaves, implants and transplants. I'll reserve my comments about their involvement with these procedures for the appropriate sections of this book.

Can They Accomplish Anything?

By encouraging their customers to shampoo frequently, they may improve scalp hygiene. If you happen to have dandruff, oily hair or an itchy scalp, proper cleansing should help—but you hardly need their products or expensive supervision to accomplish this.

The restorative treatments they offer, on the other hand,

including scalp massages, heat and ultraviolet lamps, and "special formula" lotions are nothing more than foolishness.

What Advertising Gimmicks Should You Look For?

Isolated and unrelated facts about baldness. Often these facts don't even deal with baldness but with other symptoms of hair and scalp conditions, especially those associated with dandruff.

Since dandruff may occasionally promote temporary hair loss, technically you're avoiding unnecessary shedding by controlling this condition. *But this has absolutely nothing to do with common baldness,* the problem that concerns most of these clinics' customers. Besides, if your dandruff problem is severe, you'll probably need the kind of advice or prescription that only a physician can provide. If you only have a mild case of dandruff, you should be able to control it quite easily by yourself.

The hair clinics usually do not—or cannot—explain why you are losing hair. Rather, they mix facts—or create fictions about underfed follicles or inadequate scalp circulation—to create the impression that they can do something about inherited baldness. Ideally, they should explain what kind of baldness they're attempting to treat and what they can really do about it. But if they were completely frank, they would never be able to make a customer out of you.

Personal testimonials. This sort of approach is fine for selling refrigerators, but it's worthless when dealing with medical problems. The "placebo effect"—or imagined benefits from a non-treatment—is quite common when dealing with any medical problems, including those pertaining to hair. Therefore, in any group of people receiving special "hair restorative therapy," a few are sure to think they've been helped. While they may be sincere in wanting to tell the world about it, their subjective opinions usually have no meaning for anyone else.

Before-and-after photographs. Look at figures 1 and 2 and imagine how effective they could be in a newspaper ad for a hair clinic. You can't help being impressed by the extent of the man's baldness and the completeness of his regrowth.

This man was suffering from an inflammatory condition of hair follicles known as *alopecia areata—al-lo-pé-she-ah* is the medical term for baldness, and *are á ta* means patchy. This condition, affecting perhaps one-quarter million people in this country, has no known cause, appears suddenly as one or several rounded bald spots, and may extend to leave total baldness.

The patient shown here regrew his hair because he was treated with cortisone, and only a physician can prescribe it. Occasionally, however, doing nothing may produce the same happy result—the hair may just regrow spontaneously.

Before-and-after photographs similar to these have been used by hair clinics to impress prospective customers. This type of advertising is nothing less than deceitful, because it implies a kind of therapeutic sophistication that a hair clinic could never achieve.

Why Do These Clinics Usually Offer Free Consultations?

A "free" consultation is like a "triple-your-money back" guarantee—it serves as an enticing come-on. Once you're there, they *may* misinterpret your symptoms and manipulate their examination to convince you that you have a problem that they can solve.

Meaningless comments are made concerning hair quality, bacterial and oil content of the scalp and other factors that do not relate in any significant manner to hair loss.

If a single scalp scale is found, the clinic can say you have dandruff. Since people with dandruff may lose hair temporarily,

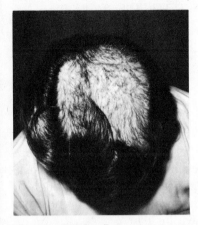

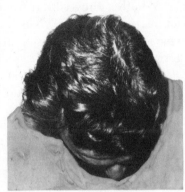

Figure 1. **"Before"**   *Figure 2.* **"After"**

This man was suffering from alopecia areata. While he may have been able to regrow his hair without medical help, his recovery was hastened by cortisone treatments that could be prescribed only by a physician.

This type of "before" and "after" picture has been used in hair "clinic" advertisements. Explanations are never offered. It is expected that the prospective customer will be so impressed by this "result," that the clinic's credibility will be instantly established—even though the clinic could never actually treat this kind of medical problem.

and since you may have dandruff, therefore, the hair you may be losing can be saved—if you're losing it from dandruff. If you think this reasoning seems a bit circular—you're right—it is!

Based on the assumption that dandruff causes shedding, if you have dandruff, the clinic can legally say they're fighting hair loss by treating your scaly scalp. Realistically, unless your scaliness is horrendous, your hair loss is probably due to other causes that they won't (and can't) inform you about.

As a general rule, getting something for nothing is usually not a bargain.

Are the Treatments Lengthy and Expensive?

Whether they vibrate your scalp, shine lights on it or rub lotions into it, your visits will probably require months or years. Many clinics try to get you to sign a contract for long-term "therapy."

As far as expense goes, at any price, the clinics have to be costly, since they actually do so little for you.

I know one man who, twenty-five years ago, spent over a thousand dollars for a course of treatments lasting several months. Today he is bald, despite those "restorative treatments" that have changed little over the years. Although he wasted his money, he felt that he would have been remiss had he not "tried everything" to save his hair.

Why Do These Clinics and Other Forms of Quackery Prosper?

Questions relating to our tolerance of all unproven types of baldness and "restorative" treatments are not easily answered.

Perhaps the answer lies in our ever-present optimism that because something needs improvement, a solution must exist somewhere.

Perhaps the quacks are clever enough to realize that most people will spend their money to be told only what they want to believe, despite all rational evidence to the contrary.

Perhaps the desire to improve ourselves overpowers our value judgments and allows us to be fooled easily. The most intelligent and clear-thinking individuals are often victimized by the most obvious flimflams when their egos are threatened. And every day, people are victimized. They may be too embarrassed to complain, or they may consider their investment in quackery too insignificant to demand retribution.

But the 50-cent vitamin capsules, the ten-dollar scalp

shampoos, and the twenty-five-dollar clinic visits add up to millions of dollars spent foolishly for promises that are rarely kept.

MAKING IT BETTER

II

Everything You Need to Know About Hair Problems

I REMEMBER A very distraught lady in her early seventies who consulted me because her scalp hair had become hopelessly thinned and unmanageable. Although she was experiencing many of the hardships associated with aging, her sense of humor remained quite vigorous: "My dentist tells me my teeth are in wonderful condition *for my age,* my eye doctor tells me my eyes are perfect *for my age* and my hairdresser tells me that my hair looks good *for my age.* But meanwhile, I have only half my teeth left, I can't see well and I can't do a thing with the little hair I have left!"

She, unfortunately, presented me with the two basic complaints that involve our scalp hair. We either worry about losing it, or we're unhappy with the way it looks.

During a lifetime, everybody will occasionally experience hair problems that fit into one or both of these categories. To deal with these difficulties, you should start with a clear understanding of why it's happening to you.

The next two chapters will provide you with practically everything you need to know about hair problems:

5. THERE MUST BE A REASON FOR YOUR HAIR LOSS.

6. WHY YOUR HAIR ISN'T WHAT YOU WANT IT TO BE.

Knowing why your hair is falling, or why it's limp or dull or unmanageable, will help you deal with the many sensible options available for either preventing or correcting these problems.

5

There Must Be a Reason for Your Hair Loss

MORE THAN NINETY percent of our skin has a hairy cover. Aside from our eyelashes, most of this hair is essentially useless. On our scalps it certainly serves no significant purpose other than adornment. Here it will grow for years—subjected to stresses as diverse as heat, moisture, sunlight, toxic chemicals, pulling, stretching, bending and other unfriendly manipulations. It will be measured and talked about, lubricated and caressed, admired or laughed at, and may even influence our personalities.

Unfortunately, some day this hair will be lost—entwined in a brush, floating in a bath tub or mysteriously unaccounted for. Its demise will somehow be noted, as it has for centuries, by the luckless individual viewing his or her thinning crown.

There *must* be a reason for your hair loss. By familiarizing yourself with the *few* conditions that create *most* of these problems, you should be able to seek the proper cosmetic or medical solutions without resorting to nonsense therapy.

The most useful way to discuss hair loss is to consider whether it occurs *permanently* or *temporarily*.

Permanent Hair Loss

Aging

As we age, hair has the unforgivable tendency to disappear from the one area we most care about—our scalps—while it flourishes in areas we couldn't care less about, such as our ears and nostrils!

When we're in our mid-teens, practically every follicle in our scalp is generating an actively growing hair. But by the time we enter our twenties, nearly every man and more than 80% of women find their hairlines receding.

As the years pass, the shedding continues. The density of our scalp hair continues to diminish. *And nobody escapes it.* An octagenarian may possess a handsome crop of scalp hair, but it must be less than he or she remembered as a teenager.

Most people accept their "aging" hair loss quite easily, since it comes about gradually. If the cosmetic deficit is slight, men tend to disregard it, while women often wear wigs for "dress-up" occasions.

Common Baldness

Common or "male-pattern" baldness affects at least 20 million Americans. We're all familiar with this condition, yet many people seek baldness "cures" when they are actually suffering from another type of hair loss, and occasionally a balding individual is shocked to learn that common baldness is the reason for his or her difficulty.

We use the term "baldness" when someone has a definite hairline recession, a "bald spot" on the crown, thinning over the top of the scalp, or combinations of any three. The sides and rear "fringe" scalp areas are usually spared, except for the inevitable thinning that accompanies age. The exact classification and the ways you can deal with this condition will be discussed in Sections IV and V.

For now, you need only remember that practically all the permanent hair loss that affects the human scalp is produced by our natural aging process and/or common baldness.

The Less-Frequent Causes of Permanent Hair Loss

They can be placed into three groups.

The first involves injury to follicles created by constant tension or pulling of scalp hair. The "pony tail" is no longer with us, but this fad left many young women with permanent bald patches on the sides of their heads. As is often the case, we've managed to find new ways to create this kind of hair loss. Tight rollers or the process of "hair weaving" may do an excellent job of killing follicles. The weaving process will be discussed in Chapter 13.

The second infrequent cause of permanent hair loss is from physical injury, such as a laceration or burn. I have seen many black women who, because they used hot irons to straighten their hair, damaged their hair follicles over the years. Hopefully, the more natural "Afro" style or the substitution of chemical straighteners will eliminate this problem.

The third cause involves various inflammatory skin disorders and growths that occasionally affect the scalp. Only one deserves mention here and that is the scalp "wen" or cyst. It tends to occur in families and requires no treatment unless it seems to be growing. Removal involves a simple office procedure and eliminates the bald spot that results from pressure of the enlarging cyst upon adjacent scalp follicles.

Temporary Hair Loss

Daily Hair Fall

Nearly everyone loses some scalp hair each day. What may become disturbing, however, is that the number of falling hairs often varies quite a bit from day to day.

No medical problem creates this daily variation in hair fall. It is *not* an abnormality, nor is the loss usually obvious to anyone but the person experiencing it.

About thirty to sixty hairs may be shed from our scalps each day. This figure, however, represents the *average* number. Days, weeks and months may pass with little to no hair fall, but nobody ever notices these delightful "quiet" interludes. Over similar time periods, large numbers of hairs may be lost, but the yearly average will remain fairly constant.

This daily variation in hair fall merely reflects the fact that our scalp follicles act independently of each other. Their three-year, three-month growth-rest cycles occur randomly. Aside from the tendency to lose more hair in the autumn, chance dictates the periods when our scalps will contain more resting hairs.

Resting hairs are the ones having the small whitish "roots" that you find in your hairbrush or bathtub. They have nowhere to go but "out."

Occasionally, hundreds of hairs may fall each day over a period of weeks to months. This kind of extreme variation is one of the most common shedding problems brought to the attention of a physician. With time, however, it always works itself out.

The "Scaly-Scalp" Conditions

Dandruff, and its two related conditions, seborrhea and

psoriasis, will be discussed in chapter 8. These "scaly-scalp" conditions may create a significant diffuse hair fall. Because they are so common, they probably account for most of the shedding that requires medical treatment. As you will learn, however, you can usually control these problems yourself.

Alopecia Areata

This condition (see chapter 4) usually produces temporary shedding of scalp—and occasionally, body—hair. In most cases, the hair either regrows spontaneously or after medical therapy. Occasionally, if this problem starts during childhood, all of the scalp and body hair may be lost permanently. Fortunately, this occurs rarely.

Pregnancy and Birth-Control Pills

Extensive shedding may follow pregnancy or discontinuation of birth-control pills (see chapter 2). After several months, the hair usually begins to regrow.

Emotional and Physical Stress

I don't believe that I have ever seen a documented case of hair loss related to *emotional* stress, unless I include the people (often youngsters) who literally pull their hair out. Too often, medical problems are blamed on "nerves," and everyone stops thinking. Most people deserve a more reasonable diagnosis, especially when the problem involves falling hair.

Hair loss can, however, be caused by *physical* stresses, although this kind of problem occurs infrequently. Years ago, typhoid fever, by raising the body temperature, often disrupted the sensitive growing follicles, throwing them into a premature resting stage. After a few months, these resting hairs were naturally shed—massively.

Today, this kind of stress hair loss is more likely to result from two other factors. I've seen patients who have lost hair because of an illness associated with a high fever (usually flu) suffered several months earlier. Another possible stress factor is a particularly difficult surgical operation. With surgery, the cause is related somehow to changes in body chemistry and not fever. Any severe illness can also create this kind of hair loss, but luckily, it does not happen too often.

Hair Breakage

This usually occurs in a woman who has had straightening, curling or bleaching improperly performed shortly before the shedding is noticed.

The offending chemicals most often producing this damage are those that can break the protein bonds within a hair, thereby permitting it to be "reshaped." Thioglycolates are the agents usually found in waving and straightening preparations. Unfortunately, they are also the active agents in chemical depilatories. Obviously, their improper use may do for the hair on your scalp what you'd prefer having done to the hair on your legs.

Peroxides, alkalies and sulfites are some of the other chemicals commonly used to change the shape and color of the hair. They, too, may have similar disastrous side effects if used improperly.

Obviously, time "cures" the problem, since the newly growing hair hasn't been affected by the chemical application.

The Less-Frequent Causes of Temporary Hair Loss

Various medications can create hair loss. The main offenders are amphetamines, blood thinners, antithyroid drugs, anti-cancer drugs (and X-ray treatments) and birth-control pills.

Hormone disorders, especially thyroid, can create a thinning problem but rarely as an isolated symptom.

Nutrition was discussed in detail in chapter 1. Aside from the crash dieters who eliminate protein from their daily supplements, nutritional deficiency is a rare cause of hair loss in this country.

The two conditions mainly responsible for creating permanent hair loss—aging and common baldness—usually develop slowly, over many years. Thinning occurs simply because the scalp follicles are no longer capable of producing new hairs.

The conditions responsible for temporary shedding usually create a thinning problem quite rapidly. Aside from hair breakage or forcible extraction, the problem is usually one of increased numbers of resting hairs, resulting often in massive hair fall.

If something occurs to double the number of resting hairs from their normal fifteen percent to thirty percent, hundreds of hairs may fall each day. If this lasts for several months, about a third of one's scalp hairs may be lost. It requires the loss of that many scalp hairs (about 30 to 40%) before thinning becomes obvious.

After the shedding abates, it may take years to return the scalp hair to its original density, since the new hair can grow only about an inch every two months.

Understanding why hair is lost should enable you to gain some insight into your own problem if one exists. Hopefully, you'll be better qualified to choose a sensible approach to correcting it either medically or cosmetically.

6

Why Your Hair Isn't What You Want It to Be

THE GREATEST CERTAINTY about hair is that everybody, at some time, will feel somewhat *uncertain* about his or her own.

The way your hair *looks* is dictated by what your parents provided for you and the environment you provide for it.

The way you *feel* about your hair is often influenced by the styles that are currently popular. When straight hair is "in," "curly-tops" become frustrated. When "frizzy" is the way to go, everyone else sulks.

Luckily, today's styling trends favor a natural look. If you understand why your hair behaves the way it does, your options are clear. You will either accept the futility of trying to change the impossible and concentrate on styling it to its fullest advantage, or you will direct yourself to the corrective measures that can make a difference.

To enable you to make these sensible choices, you should understand why your hair looks the way it does. I've categorized the physical attributes of hair into:

SHAPE AND SIZE
TEXTURE
COLOR
MANAGEABILITY
GROWTH

DENSITY
"WEATHERING"

Shape and Size—Your Follicles Are at the Root of It.

Why Hair Is Straight or Curly

The degree of curliness of a hair seems to relate directly to the curvature of the follicle that produces it. Hairs are composed of individual fibers that are deposited upon each other. If a follicle is curved, the "inside" fibers are squeezed closer together than those on the outer edge.

The emerging hair reflects the shape of its follicle exactly. Physicians performing hair transplants are quite familiar with this phenomenon. When removing a graft from a curly-haired scalp, they know that the cut must be angled quite carefully to avoid piercing the curved follicles. Despite claims to the contrary, there is no way that cutting hair should make it turn from straight to curly or visa versa.

Hair retains its shape because its fibers are "cemented" to their neighbors by protein bonds that can be broken only by excessive heat or certain chemicals. When hair is straightened or curled, its new shape is held together by new protein bonds.

You should never forget that your hairs are not as "solid" as they appear but, rather, are intricate networks of fibers connected by chemical "bridges." Their shape can be changed, but not repeatedly (see chapter 10). If these protein bonds are broken once too often, they may not re-form and their hairs break.

Why Hair Is Fine or Coarse

As hair shape relates to the curvature of its follicle, hair size relates directly to the size of its follicle.

Larger follicles produce thicker hairs. During the first decade of our lives, our scalp follicles become larger with each new
hair cycle. These hairs, in turn, possess increasingly larger
diameters, until, by about age twelve, our scalps contain only
adult-size hairs.

The "adult-size" of a follicle varies. Many young adults have
very fine scalp hair associated with perfectly mature, though
smaller, follicles. With increasing age, however, many people
discover that their hair not only becomes thinned out, but
what's left is often finer. Interestingly, senile follicles actually
become more juvenile—their smaller size means finer hair.

Unlike shape, hair size cannot really be changed. Even
coating agents accomplish little for fine hair, and coarse hair can
be thinned "out" but not "down." Cutting hair never thickens
it. This myth is probably derived from the teenager who starts
shaving when his beard is naturally thickening and the woman
who, after shaving her legs, is left with a coarse stubble unlike
the finely tapered new hairs that regrow after waxing.

Since the size of your hair is determined by the anatomy of
your follicles, you cannot alter what's already there, but you can
create an illusion of thicker hair by enhancing its manageability
through conditioning (chapter 9), "body waving," bleaching
and tinting (chapter 10), and proper styling (chapter 11).

Texture—"Normal" Hair Is Easy to Cultivate

By "texture," I mean the *natural* dryness or oiliness of your
hair, unrelated to the effects of environment or improper use of
grooming aids.

We usually relate the condition of hair to the activity—or
inactivity—of the scalp's oil glands.

In some dandruff-producing disorders, the scalp and hair

are often quite dry because the oil glands are either underactive due to inflammation or their oil cannot flow properly when the accumulated scales block the follicle openings.

In acne and related conditions, the oil glands may become so overactive that the accumulated grease covers the scalp and mats down the hair.

Since most of us are not troubled by these problems, we should be enjoying normal scalps and hair. How "normal" translates into oil gland activity is not as obvious as many cosmetologists will have you believe. For example, infants, young children and many women possess very small—and essentially inactive—oil glands. Yet their scalps and hair are as "normal" as anyone might hope for.

The lesson you should learn from this is that you needn't bother with the brushing, massaging, oil treatments, vitamins and other foolishness that promises to make your oil glands work better. Instead, concentrate your efforts on maintaining a healthy scalp by proper cleansing (chapters 7 and 8). If your scalp and hair are still too dry or oily, you probably need the kind of advice and care that only a dermatologist can dispense.

Color—It's Locked In

The pigment responsible for hair color is called *melanin*. It's contained in tiny granules that are "locked into" the hair shaft beneath its covering layer or cuticle. Differences in the chemical structure of melanin account for the variation in natural hair color that ranges from black to red to blond. A graying scalp contains a mixture of partially pigmented and white hairs. A white hair simply contains no melanin.

The only way in which hair color can be changed is by bleaching or dyeing (chapter 10). No physical manipulation can alter hair color—"pull out one gray hair, get seven"—nor is it possible for pigmented hairs to suddenly "turn white overnight."

People have "turned white" suddenly but for a different reason. They were suffering from alopecia areata, that medical condition capable of creating rapid, massive hair fall (chapter 4). For reasons unknown, white hairs are more resistent. Someone who has "gray" hair might lose the darker ones suddenly, be left with all of his or her white hair, and appear to have "turned white overnight."

Manageability—Look Around You

If you've come to terms with your scalp and it's neither dry nor oily, doesn't itch or shed scales, and your hair still is limp or "flying away"—look around you.

When you check out your environment, you'll realize that it's often too dry or wet, or it's composed of air that the weathermen euphemistically call "unacceptable" rather than "polluted."

The relative humidity of the air dictates how "dry" or "wet" your hair may feel. The protein that makes up hair—and skin—has an affinity for water. This phenomenon has been made obvious to anyone whose skin has become white and swollen after being immersed in water. During periods of low humidity, such as the wintertime, our skin becomes chapped because the dry air literally pulls out its water.

Hair, composed of a similar water-loving protein, reacts similarly to changes in the environment. When the air is dry, hairs lose their water to the surrounding air, and they become dry. Dry hairs build up a negative static electric charge that causes them to repel their neighbors, creating the problem of "fly-away." When the air is "wet," hairs soak up the water, swell and tend to sag under their own weight—or become "limp."

The pollutants present in air that has become increasingly

"unacceptable" are caught by our scalp hairs and adhere to their oily surfaces. The hairs lose their "body," becoming limp, and lose their normal texture, becoming "dull."

These problems can be handled quite easily by changing the frequency of your cleansing schedules (chapter 7) and finding the proper conditioning agents (chapter 9).

Growth–Rapunzel Was a Fake!

"My hair just doesn't grow." This may be quite true but, normally, only for the fifteen percent of our scalp hairs that have entered their resting phase. Since these resting hairs are scattered diffusely, throughout our scalps, it seems rather unlikely that they could be noticed easily enough to account for this common complaint.

People may imagine that their scalp hair *isn't* growing, because they usually don't understand how slowly hair actually *does* grow. I have often thought that some individuals expect to see their hairs lengthen if they look closely enough—sort of a "Rapunzel complex."

Hair grows only about one-half inch per month. Since its growing time averages between two and six years, it's maximum attainable length averages between one and three feet. Some people do have faster growing hair, and some hair may grow for as long as eight years. At that rate, a hair might reach almost four feet, but that would be an exceptional size. I would expect that to have ankle-length hair, you'd have to be quite short!

Does enough hair ever stop growing in any scalp area so that we might easily notice it? This may occur in the late stages of common baldness or earlier, when a hairline starts to recede.

Hair follicles, in their final days, have very short growth and very long resting cycles. A hair having a shortened growth period becomes a short hair. Since this same hair will have a resting period lasting for months or years, it will remain atop the head without growing until it finally falls out.

This accounts for the short wispy hairs seen on a receding hairline or a bald head. They are the hairs we notice that simply "don't grow."

Healthy hair follicles, on the other hand, will continue to provide new hairs even if their growing hairs are accidentally or purposely plucked. The old-wives' tale that tweezing kills follicles is simply a falsehood.

The way your hair grows—or doesn't grow—is controlled by the kind of follicles you've inherited. The patterns for growth and structure were "programmed" before you entered this world. (chapter 16).

Complaints about hair growth are the most difficult to deal with. Look to your stylist (chapter 11) to help you keep what's there looking good.

Density–Whether Your Hair Is "Thick" or "Thin"

Complaints about "thin," or sparsely distributed scalp hair often accompany those of "non-growing" hair. Once again, the responsible factor relates to the way in which you've inherited your follicles.

If your follicles have endowed you with blond hairs, you can expect them in numbers reaching 150,000. Redheads will count the lowest numbers of scalp hairs—around 100,000—while brunets are in between.

While your hair's color correlates with its density, you may, of course, find it thinning for any of the reasons discussed in chapter 5. If your change from "thick" to "thin" is permanent, refer to the chapters describing hair management in section III and hair replacement in sections IV and V.

"Weathering"–The Ways We Damage Our Hair

A single strand of hair stands up remarkably well under the self-inflicted and environmental stresses we place upon it. From the time it sprouts, it may serve us for years, in nearly mint condition. But, things do go wrong.

Damage Directed Against the Hair Cuticle

Most damage is directed against the cuticle, or hair surface. Sunlight, water and many of our aggressive grooming aids eventually take their toll by destroying this protective covering.

The cuticle consists of a layered series of flattened rings that encircle the hair shaft. Each covers the one beneath it and is placed slightly forward so that in cross section, a hair is covered by several protective layers.

Figure 3 shows this layering effect of the cuticle. This is the way it should look—and usually does on the portion of a hair closest to the scalp.

After a hair has been growing for about a year, its cuticle begins to lift off and fragment (Figure 4).

By the time a hair is two to three years old, its ends begin to fray, even if it has been carefully managed. If it grows long enough, it eventually loses part or all of the cuticle covering its end, and it splits. Figure 5 shows these irregular bundles of hair fibers that protrude from the tip of a hair, creating the "split end."

This progressive degeneration of a hair's protective cuticle is referred to as "weathering." Most of the ways we usually damage our hair are directed against the cuticle:

- Shampoos that are too alkaline tend to make the edges of the cuticle lift off the hair surface.
- Sunlight, blow-drying, bleaching, dyeing, straightening

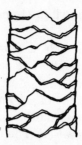

Figure 3. This illustrates the appearance of the hair surface magnified 1,000 times. The cuticle actually consists of flattened rings, resembling roof shingles except that they encircle the hair shaft.

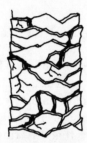

Figure 4. The cuticle is seen several inches from the scalp representing the portion of a hair that is about a year old. The cuticle has broken into smaller fragments that have begun to stand away from the hair shaft.

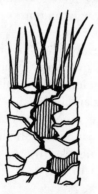

Figure 5. The tip of the hair has lost its cuticle. Irregular bundles of hair fibers protrude to create the "split end."

and backcombing contribute to premature fracture of the cuticle.

- Extreme measures, such as over-bleaching or teasing, may create more penetrating damage resulting in hair breakage.

When the cuticle is no longer intact, its hair becomes tangled and dull. Wool is an example of a hair naturally possessing cuticle edges that are raised. The fiber, therefore, appears dull and is easily woven (tangled).

The use of special conditioning agents may temporarily improve the quality of "weathered" hair (chapter 9).

Damage Directed Against the Hair Shaft

Hair may occasionally be damaged from within, rather than by agents that attack its surface.

Since hair is a product of an active organ—the follicle—its well-being relates directly to an individual's general state of health. In the same way that the rings of a tree trunk often reflect past stresses, a hair may provide its own "record" by developing constrictions within its shaft.

- A hair's diameter may become diminished during periods of illness. If severe enough, an illness may even create premature hair fall (chapter 5).
- Malnutrition, especially when involving protein deficiency, may induce similar problems (chapter 1).

Advice about maintaining the health of your hair through proper eating, sleeping and exercising is well taken, but these factors usually operate in a negative manner. Doing the wrong things may create hair damage or shedding, but doing *more* of the right things won't necessarily make your hair any better than nature intended it to be.

You should now understand why your hair looks the way it does, why it may fall out and why you should avoid the foolishness that underlies most hair restoration schemes. With this background, you should be better prepared to understand and evaluate the various methods available for making your hair look better or for replacing it if it's gone.

III

Making the Most of What You Have

"WHAT SHAMPOO SHOULD I BUY, and how often should I use it?"

"My dandruff drives me crazy!"

"How can I control my frizzies, fly-away, split ends?"

"Should I perm it, wave it, color it?"

"How should I style it?"

Our interest in hair has become something of a national fetish. In 1975, we spent $632,320,000 for shampoos, $313,910,000 for hair coloring, $358,940,000 for hair dressings, conditioners, rinses, permanents and other styling aids, and $300,070,000 for hair sprays—and incidentally, $17,190,000 for depilatories to remove some of it. The fact that we spend over one and one-half billion dollars a year, just for products to groom what we have atop our heads, certainly indicates that we care.

Now that you understand why your hair problems exist, you're ready to start solving them. There's something out there for everyone—whether you have too little hair or hair that is simply unmanageable.

The advertising industry has performed a commendable service in calling our attention to the many grooming and styling aids available today. Their flowery descriptions, however, often tend to confuse rather than clarify what these products are supposed to accomplish.

I'll try to erase some of this mumbo jumbo in the five chapters devoted to hair care:

Advertising aside, the cosmetic industry has provided us with enough preparations to meet most of our reasonable requirements, and their products are usually both elegant and honest. We needn't take many of their claims too seriously. After all, my daughter does love her assorted fruit-flavored rinses, and my son (and I) couldn't be happier with his Mickey Mouse shampoo dispenser.

7

Shampoos

ABOUT THREE HUNDRED YEARS AGO, a cosmetic discovery was made that revolutionized our habits. Fatty acid soaps were introduced and people really began to clean themselves.

Until the 1940's, soaps remained unchallenged as our basic cleansing agent. During those years, as newly developed synthetic detergents were marketed, soaps lost popularity. Today, it is difficult to find a commercial soap shampoo.

The synthetic detergents succeeded because our hair required shampoos that had to cope with newer and more sophisticated problems.

The "dirt" we found clinging to our hair consisted not only of natural scalp scales and oil, but of new kinds of environmental particles and a host of new cosmetic chemicals.

Additionally, our shampoos were required to "prepare" our hair so that our newer styling and grooming aids could perform their jobs properly.

The $600 million-plus spent yearly on shampoos represents a product selection that is dazzling and—to many people— often confusing. But don't despair. Since most are quite good, your chances of finding a satisfactory product are excellent.

Aren't Detergent Shampoos Bad for Hair?

The most oft-quoted myth concerning cleansing products is

that soaps, being derived from natural sources, are somehow superior to synthetic detergents that may harm our hair.

While soaps are *derived* from animal fats or vegetable oils, in order to work, they must first be *synthetically* modified with alkalis. "Surfactant" is the name given to man-made chemicals that do exactly what man-*changed* soaps do—they cleanse. Moreover, they may not only be as effective as soaps, they may be even *milder.*

The word "detergent" refers to any cleansing agent, whether it is derived from natural sources (soaps) or synthetically-combined chemicals (surfactants).

If you try to avoid detergent shampoos, you'll have nothing available with which to wash your hair. If you eliminate synthetic detergents, you'll probably have to make your own soap shampoo.

Why Aren't Soap Shampoos Popular Today?

The major reason is that our water simply isn't soft enough for soap. The calcium and magnesium salts, which create water "hardness," combine with soap to leave a sticky dull film or "scum" over hair, which, while clean, becomes "lifeless" or "unmanageable."

Modern detergent shampoos, however, work well in hard water and rinse out completely.

What Else Does a Shampoo Contain?

Aside from a cleansing agent (detergent), it contains (mostly) water. The usual additives consist of foaming agents to create the lather that isn't really necessary for cleansing, opacifiers and thickeners to enhance cosmetic acceptability and coloring and fragrance to provide product "identity."

Are There Cancer-Producing Agents in Shampoos?

Recently, a fairly weak cancer-producing agent belonging to a group of chemicals known as nitrosamines has been identified in many cosmetic preparations, including some commercial shampoos.

The nitrosamine is not added to these products, but is found as a by-product from reactions between other chemicals. While this agent has produced liver cancer in rats, its effects upon humans are still unclear.

Cosmetic companies are trying to eliminate this contaminant from their products. They do point out, however, that nitrosamines are usually present in the air in high concentrations, and they can be formed by the body after foods such as bacon, tomato, spinach and bread are eaten. In fact, the natural nitrosamine formation within our bodies may be greater than the direct exposure from *all* outside sources.

How Does a Shampoo Work?

The combination of a detergent, warm water and massaging action removes dirt and natural scales along with cosmetic and natural oils from hair.

The cleansing process is both mechanical and chemical.

What Are Dry Shampoos?

They usually consist of absorbent powders and mild alkalis. An alkali can chemically remove some oily residue, while a powder physically binds the loosened "dirt." They certainly do not represent a choice method for cleansing hair, but they are useful when regular shampooing is impossible, as during periods of illness.

How Do Shampoos Damage Hair?

Since detergents cannot differentiate between natural oils and environmental dirt, shampoos may dry hair too severely, creating "fly-away."

Stronger cleansing depends upon alkalinity, which may cause the edges of the hair cuticle to lift off, creating dull surface texture and tangles.

By introducing milder detergents or by decreasing alkalinity, a shampoo's cleansing action can be made less aggressive and therefore, less damaging. "Squeaky-clean" hair is probably "over-cleansed" hair. It is not usually necessary or desirable.

Do "Acid Balanced" Shampoos Avoid These Problems?

They do, but don't worry too much about finding one, since most shampoos marketed today are "acid balanced."

Someone, many years ago, innocently coined the phrase "acid mantle" to describe the surface of the skin and hair, which is thought to be slightly acidic.

While I won't argue with the fact that a highly alkaline substance such as lye will damage hair and skin protein, so will the other extreme, a strong acid, do the same. The safest range for a detergent is around neutral. Even the strongest alkaline shampoo sold today is milder than the average bar of soap.

Since most modern detergent shampoos are formulated around the neutral range, the advertising claims that flaunt this fact are simply unnecessary.

How Important Are Conditioner Additives for Preventing Hair Damage?

Although I usually dislike "combination" products, conditioners added to shampoos probably help to prevent some hair damage. Whether they're protein derivatives or other forms of "hair builders," they all seem to reduce split ends, dullness and tangling to some extent.

Your shampoo should probably be chosen for its cleansing properties and not its potential for repairing damaged hair. Enough post-shampoo conditioners are available for that purpose.

Can Shampooing Too Often Make Your Hair Fall Out?

This question represents the classic old-wives' tale concerning scalp hygiene.

Resting hairs—or hairs that have finished growing and are ready to fall—are always present on an adult scalp. Estimates of shedding run as high as 100 to 150 hairs a day, although 30 to 60 are probably closer to the average number.

Shampooing, brushing or simply pulling will hasten their departure by a day or two. The point is, they're going to fall out anyway, so losing them a little sooner is of no significant import.

By delaying your scalp cleansing, you merely fool yourself by keeping these hairs in place a while longer. It's not worth the sacrifice, because they only build up and *appear* to fall out in greater numbers when you postpone your shampoo for many days or weeks.

If you shampoo once every two weeks, you'll simply harvest a fourteen-day supply of resting hairs and achieve nothing more than a dirty scalp.

How Often Should You Shampoo?

I advise most people to try to shampoo as often as possible—*daily,* in most cases.

Your frequency of shampooing should depend upon the amount of oil you naturally secrete, the quantity of dirt your environment deposits on your scalp, the season of the year and your styling requirements.

- A mechanic will obviously require more frequent scalp cleansing than an infant.
- Summer athletic activities that make your head sweat may require shampooing several times a day, while winter inactivity and dry air may enable you to skip two or three days.
- The woman receiving her weekly wash in a beauty parlor may complain about itchy scalp, dandruff and "lifeless" hair, but it's the cross she must bear if she's unwilling to shampoo between visits.

In general, you should shampoo as often as necessary to keep your scalp and hair feeling and looking good. I would estimate a reasonable frequency to number between daily and once every three days. The number of times you lather during each shampoo depends upon how dirty or oily your hair seems. Usually, when you are shampooing often, one lathering is adequate.

How Should You Evaluate Your Shampoo Needs?

Dryness or Oiliness of Your Scalp

Dry scalps tend to itch and flake, while dry hair is difficult to keep in place—it "flies away."

Oily scalps usually produce oily hair which feels that way several hours after shampooing. Such hair looks greasy and mats down. Running your fingers over it or rubbing it with a dry cloth usually deposits an oily film. This type of problem is often associated with an oily complexion or acne.

Normal scalp and hair usually feels and looks good for a day or two after shampooing. The hair is soft and has a slightly oily surface. Moreover, it retains its "body" and neither flies away nor mats down.

Season of the Year

On a cold winter day, the relative humidity, particularly indoors, may drop to ten or fifteen per cent. Skin and hair, however, feel and look good with a humidity of about sixty per cent. Under adverse winter conditions, a normal scalp and hair will lose its water to the air and dry out. Milder shampoos used less often may be helpful.

During the hot humid days of summer, especially if you're active, your hair may swell and mat down because it absorbs water from the atmosphere and your own sweat secretions. Salt crystallizing out from your sweat and environmental dirt may stick to your hair diminishing its sheen. A normal scalp and hair may require more frequent washing with your regular shampoo or a stronger product.

Use of Grooming Aids

Bleaching, dyeing, straightening and perming may damage the hair's cuticle creating surface cracks that make shampoos formulated for "normal" hair difficult to use. Products with added conditioners will probably work better and may even protect the more fragile "treated" hairs from the mechanical damage induced by shampooing, combing, brushing and hot-air drying.

Hair sprays and other dressings often leave deposits on hair making it dull and "lifeless." Stronger shampoos used more frequently may be beneficial.

The Type of Hair You Have and the Way You Style It.

Longer hair may develop more split ends. Conditioning shampoos may help.

Short layered cuts will require frequent shampooing to keep the hair dry enough to maintain its body.

Thin, fine hair also requires more shampooing and conditioning to keep its body.

Coarse thick hair may actually demand more gentle shampoos in order to leave natural oils in place to keep it more manageable.

Your Work and Athletic Activities

More environmental dirt and sweat will require more frequent and stronger shampoos.

Hardness of Your Water

Unless you wash your hair with soap, this should not be a problem, since most commercial shampoos work well in the hardest water.

Related Scalp Conditions

Dandruff and other scaly scalp problems will be discussed in the next chapter.

What Should a Shampoo Do for You?

It should, of course, cleanse your hair and scalp. Any excessive oiliness, scaliness or environmental or cosmetic "dirt" should be removed.

It should rinse out easily.

It should leave your hair manageable and looking good. If your hair still mats or appears dull, try a new shampoo. If your hair is clean but flies away, try a conditioner.

It should possess a pleasant fragrance, because your hair will probably retain its scent for at least a few hours. If you want to smell like a fruit salad, at least pick a flavor that you enjoy eating. But beware of scents that may attract bees and other insects, especially if you're allergic to them.

It should be easy to use. If liquid, try to find a product that uses a dispenser, instead of a screw top, to avoid spillage.

It should always be reasonably priced. Bargain shampoos, by the way, are not always as economical as they claim, because they are often quite diluted and require larger quantities for proper cleansing.

Should You Brush Vigorously Before Shampooing to Loosen Dirt? Should You Massage Your Shampoo into Your Scalp in a Prescribed Manner to Stimulate Circulation?

No.

Suggestions of Shampoos Available for Various Types of Scalps and Hair.

If you were to purchase every commercial shampoo available at the moment you're reading this, and if you used a different product each day, it would take about two years to try them all. Moreover, by the time you finished, you probably would have to start all over again, because during that two-year period, a whole slew of new products would have been marketed.

Another difficulty inherent in suggesting shampoos concerns something that dermatologists have always been aware of and that *Consumer Reports* in their November, 1976 issue on shampoos stated quite succinctly: that "common sense doesn't seem to have much to do with shampoos."

They discovered that, among other things, men and women do not usually like the same shampoo, that fragrance influences personal preference, and that people seem to choose shampoos that they aren't supposed to like. For example, people with oily hair more often preferred "dry hair" shampoos and vice versa.

Notwithstanding these formidable obstacles, I'll offer suggestions of several products that should be useful for varying types of scalps and hair. I've compiled this list based on the *Consumer Reports* testing, marketing figures for popular shampoos, and my patients' and my own personal preferences.

Where pertinent, I'll note whether the product is male or female oriented. I've eliminated the so-called "price" shampoos, i.e., the cheaper private label products sold in supermarkets, because as I mentioned earlier, they're often diluted and not the bargains they appear to be. I will not list any "luxury" products, because they tend to be ridiculously over-priced and offer nothing over the popular commercial brands except fancy packaging.

Most shampoos formulated for general usage are in liquid, gel or cream form. Other types useful for specific problems include concentrated, conditioning and baby shampoos. The products are listed alphabetically.

NORMAL HAIR AND SCALP, assuming a temperate "spring-autumn" climate and a "clean" occupation.

For Men	For Women
Danex	Avon Hi-Lite, Normal
Halo, Normal	Breck Basic Texturizing
Head & Shoulders, Cream	with Protein
Herbal Essence, Delicate	Danex
Lemon Up	Everynight, Lemon
Prell Concentrate	Head & Shoulders, Cream
New Alberto VO-5	Herbal Essence, Delicate
Suave, Green Apple	Prell Concentrate
VO-5, Normal	Revlon Flex Balsam &
Wella Care Herbal, Liquid	Protein, Concentrate
Yucca-dew, Normal	Revlon Milk Plus 6,
	Normal to Dry
	Suave, Lemon
	Wella Herbal Blossoms,
	Normal

OILY HAIR AND SCALP. Also NORMAL HAIR with excess environmental and cosmetic "dirt" or requiring "extra" cleansing due to high humidity and sweat accumulation.

For Men	For Women
Avon Hi-Lite, Oily	Alberto Balsam, Oily
Head & Shoulders, Cream	Head & Shoulders, Cream
Ionax	Ionax
Pernox	Pernox
Prell Concentrate	Prell Concentrate
Wella Care Herbal,	Wella Herbal Blossoms, Oily
Concentrate	Zincon
Zincon	

EXCESSIVELY OILY HAIR AND SCALP that may be caused by seborrhea. (see chapter 8).

DRY HAIR AND SCALP. Also VERY FINE AND VERY
COARSE "TREATED" HAIR, or hair that is dull, splitting
and/or "lifeless" due to excessive bleaching, dyeing, straightening, perming or environmental exposure.

For Men

Breck Gold Formula, Dry	Mennen Baby Magic
DHS	Protein 21, Dry
Herbal Essence, Delicate	Wella Balsam
Johnson's Baby	

For Women

Breck Baby	Lustre-Creme Conditioning
Breck Basic Texturizing	Protein 21, Dry
with Protein	Revlon Flex Balsam &
DHS	Protein concentrated
Earth Born Baby	Revlon 'Milk Plus 6',
Earth Born, Dry, Avocado	Normal to Dry
Herbal Essence, Delicate	Wella Herbal Blossoms, Dry
Johnson's Baby	

These listings do not reflect my endorsement of any of these
products over others that may be as good. They merely represent a sampling of shampoos that seem to please a majority of
people using them for their specific types of scalp and hair. You
certainly should try several brands before choosing favorites.
Additionally, you should probably stock a few shampoos in your
medicine cabinet, since most people seem to tire of any product after constant use.

8

Controlling Dandruff

DANDRUFF IS characterized by two consistent features—practically everybody gets it and nobody knows how to cure it.

It is so common to all of us that its frequency need not be verified by any statistical study, although several years ago a "dandruff poll" revealed that 94 per cent of people questioned said they experienced the problem at some time.

No "disease label" has ever been pinned on dandruff, although there has never been a lack of "theories" available to explain it. The blame has shifted from scalp bacteria to hormone production, to oil gland malfunction or to other factors that might suggest that dandruff is something other than an undesirable human condition that remains incurable, but is certainly controllable.

What Is Dandruff?

If you discover fine white scales flaking off your scalp and it isn't hair spray, you probably have dandruff. It's important to note that this condition does not produce any redness, swelling, or scabbing of scalps, although mild itching may be associated with it.

"False" and "True" Dandruff

Both types look alike, but their causes differ.

"False" dandruff is related to improper scalp hygiene. Skin naturally scales because it turns itself over every 28 days. The flaking surface cells combine to form visible scales that are not usually obvious because bathing and accidental rubbing remove them.

The hairs present on a neglected scalp act as a magnet for those scales if they haven't been shampooed or brushed away. Frequent cleansing easily solves this kind of problem.

The "true" dandruff that has plagued so many of us may begin as early as our fifth year, becoming commonplace during our teens. While its exact cause is still a mystery, it seems to result from a slight increase in the normal 28-day turnover of skin. The success of antiseptic shampoos suggests that scalp bacteria or chemicals produced by their activity may contribute to a scalp's tendency to scale.

Will Sterilizing Combs and Brushes Improve or Prevent a Dandruff Problem?

No. The bacteria growing on a scalp's surface—or any other area of skin—belong there. While it is certainly possible for a contaminated comb or brush to introduce infection-producing bacteria or fungi, your own grooming instruments should not normally require any other care aside from occasional soap and water cleansings.

The Other Scaly Scalp Conditions

Several skin disorders may create a scaly scalp problem which may erroneously be called dandruff.

Seborrhea (*seb' o-ré ah*), an inflammatory disorder of oil

glands, usually affects the scalp, which begins to produce scales that are usually thicker and more abundant than those found in dandruff. The scaling, either patchy or diffuse, arises from a scalp that is reddened because of the underlying oil gland inflammation.

The control of this disorder, extremely common in people between the ages of twenty to forty, may require prescription medication along with therapeutic dandruff shampoos.

Psoriasis *(so-ri' ah-sis)*, affecting several million Americans, may produce large quantities of scale because the affected skin turns over ten times more rapidly than normal. Like seborrhea, it is associated with inflammation which translates into reddened—and perhaps swollen—skin patches. Again, treatment provides only control rather than cure. Most people suffering from psoriasis will require medical advice.

Ringworm and other skin disorders may also create scalp scaliness. Because they usually do not respond to non-prescription medications, these problems eventually receive proper medical attention.

Do Any of the Scaly Scalp Conditions Produce Hair Loss?

Interestingly, people with severe psoriasis may not complain of any increased hair fall, while those with mild dandruff may swear they're losing sinksfull.

If you have dandruff, seborrhea or psoriasis, and you're experiencing increased hair fall because of one of these conditions, remember that this kind of shedding is both temporary and reversible, and *not* related in any way to common baldness. The falling hairs are often those broken by excessive rubbing and scratching. They should all regrow after the scaling problem is brought under control.

How Is Hair and Scalp Affected by These Conditions?

When *dandruff* is present, the affected scalp is usually dry and often itchy. The hair may feel dry or normal. During the warmer summer months, both scalp and hair may become more oily since gland activity usually increases with higher temperatures.

Seborrhea usually implies oiliness. People often complain of excessively greasy scalps and hair because of this condition. When scaly patches begin to build up over the scalp, it may begin to itch and feel dry along with the hair.

When large scalp areas are affected by *psoriasis* or severe seborrhea, the scales occlude the follicle openings blocking the natural flow of oil, resulting in both dry hair and scalp.

What Factors Aggravate These Conditions?

Dandruff, if not related to improper scalp hygiene, seems to have few known causes. Winter dryness may increase skin and scalp scaliness while the tendency to shampoo less often during that season may encourage the scales to accumulate.

Seborrhea is occasionally triggered by emotional and dietary stress—the latter involving "stimulants" such as alcohol, caffeine and spicy foods.

Psoriasis can also be flared by emotional stress, but dietary factors, while frequently suggested, seem to have little influence on either inciting or improving this condition.

While it would be useful to understand what factors, if any, can make your scalp scale, most people cannot usually offer any reason for flare-ups of these conditions.

Controlling Dandruff

If you're not suffering from the "false" dandruff of neglect, and you've been cleansing often with the proper product for your type of hair and scalp, and you're still troubled by scaliness, you should next try one of the so-called "therapeutic" shampoos. The schedules outlined below should work for dandruff and *mild* seborrhea or psoriasis.

Try one product for several days. If you're not improved, switch to a new one from another group. If, after shampooing daily for a week or two, you still haven't noted enough improvement, add a pre-shampoo treatment to your daily regimen.

Remember that these suggestions apply only to the mild scaly scalp conditions discussed in this chapter. Any problem that fails to respond should certainly be checked by a physician. Many a case of scalp lice has been unsuccessfully treated as "dandruff" before it was finally noticed that some of the "scales" had legs!

The effective therapeutic shampoos that may be purchased over the counter fall into four groups. They are listed alphabetically and include the popular brands.

I would suggest starting with one product from each of the first three groups, shampooing daily with it for a few days, then changing to one of the other products for a few more days. *Chances are that no matter how effective a particular shampoo seems to be, it will lose its effectiveness after continued use.* "Switching around" usually solves this problem. When you "switch back" to a previously-used product, it often seems to regain its original effectiveness.

Most of these shampoos require an initial wash followed by a second lathering which is left on the scalp for several minutes before being rinsed off.

Group 1. Sulfur-Salicylic Acid shampoos gently peel the surface layers of scalp to aid scale removal.
Fostex
Ionil
Meted
Sebulex, cream or liquid
Vanseb

Group 2. Tar shampoos usually add the tar to a sulfur-salicylic acid product to provide a mild anti-inflammatory effect.
DHS Tar
Icon (gel)
Ionil T
Pentrax
Polytar
Sebutone, cream or liquid
Tersa-tar
Vanseb-T

Group 3. Zinc Pyrithione shampoos work better than the shampoo base without this mild antiseptic agent, perhaps by decreasing the amount or activity of scalp bacteria and/or irritants they produce.
Danex
Head & Shoulders, cream and liquid
Zincon

Group 4. Selenium Sulfide shampoos work, but how they work is not known. They are sold by prescription only, but one "half-strength" product is sold over the counter: Selsun Blue.

Supplemental Regimens

Pre-Shampoo Treatment

These products may be applied to the scalp and left on for up to several hours, to loosen scales and/or to treat mild seborrhea or psoriasis. They should be used sparingly and washed out well.

Diasporal cream
P & S liquid
Pragmatar

Oil Turban

This "treatment" may be effective in treating persistent scaling. With certain substitutions for prescription products, I often use this for severe seborrheal or psoriatic scaling.
1. Wash with tar shampoo.
2. Rub in olive, mineral, or commercial bath oil.
3. Wet 2 towels in hot water and wrap around scalp.
4. Cover towels with a plastic shower cap.
5. Remove in ½ hour.
6. Shampoo with product from Group 1, 3, or 4.
7. Rub in a post-shampoo product if desired.

Post-Shampoo Treatment

These are mildly active anti-seborrheic treatments that can be left in the scalp after shampooing. They may also help an itchy scalp.

Drest, hair dressing (antiseptic)
Sebucare, hair dressing (mild peeling effect)
Top Brass, hair dressing (antiseptic)

You should be able to control most minor dandruff problems with only a few of these shampoos or supplemental regimens. Additionally, you should avoid excessive use of hair sprays or other grooming aids that tend to "cake up" on hair.

If any scalp irritation develops, stop using the offending product completely and hold off using any therapeutic product until the irritation subsides.

Tar may impart a yellowish stain to grey or blond hair.

Selenium sulfide overuse has been reported to produce hair discoloration or "greasiness."

Overuse of any of these shampoos or pre-shampoo products could create a dry scalp.

In general, all these products work well and are safe to use often. Be prepared to vary your treatment schedules with the natural fluctuations of your dandruff problem.

9

Conditioners

UNTIL I BECAME A dermatologist, the only "split end" I ever thought about ran with a football. This term now evokes an image of another way that hair becomes ravaged by the effects of grooming aids, environment, and its natural aging process.

Luckily, hair is forgiving. No matter how we damage it, new strands continue to appear. Because it grows at the leisurely rate of about an inch every two months, what we have available must be kept looking good.

Since most hair damage usually affects the surface layers, temporary correction can be accomplished with conditioners. Today we need not depend upon lemon juice, vinegar, beer and raw eggs, but rather we can choose from hundreds of elegant preparations that are quite easy to use.

Whatever type of conditioning agent you require, it will probably be applied to your hair *after* you shampoo. In fact, since dirt inhibits its action, proper shampooing is essential.

How Do Conditioners Help Hair?

Each of the six types of conditioners that I've listed below performs one or several of four tasks.
- It may flatten the hair cuticle to enhance sheen.
- It may reduce "fly-away."
- It may contain "body builders" that further enhance sheen,

repair surface cracks or even penetrate the hair shaft to increase "body."

- It may contain agents that coat the hair to "set" it in place.

How Often Are Conditioners Needed?

They should be used as often as necessary to correct the kind of damage for which they've been formulated. For example, hair that normally looks good without conditioning may need it daily when the weather is hot, dry and sunny.

Can They Harm Hair?

No. They are quite safe. If, however, they are used too often or for the wrong kind of hair, they may coat and mat hair down, creating a "greasy" look.

Types of Conditioners

The first four types that I'll describe encompass all of the products that are called "conditioners." They are massaged into hair after shampooing and are usually rinsed out after a variable period of time. Each succeeding type evolved from the one before and is chemically more complex.

The final two types are applied after shampooing and are not rinsed out. They are basically setting preparations, but they tend to condition in the sense that they add body to hair.

Again, I'll list several products alphabetically. Unless noted, they can be used by either sex. I've avoided naming any luxury products, because they seem to differ from the popularly priced brands only by virtue of their packaging.

The Acid Rinse

This is the original and simplest type of conditioning agent. If you're on a natural cosmetic kick, you might try equal parts of lemon juice and water or six parts of vinegar diluted with one part of water. They are massaged into the hair after a shampoo and rinsed out.

Acid rinses condition only by removing any "scum" or film left on hair by soap or any other highly alkaline cleanser. They act by re-flattening the hair's cuticle to permit whatever *natural* sheen you possess to show. They are not anti-static, so "fly-away" will not be prevented.

Since most commercial shampoos are not highly alkaline, the acid rinse has more historical significance than practical value.

Creme Rinse Conditioners

If your hair is naturally dull, or dull and tangly because your hair's cuticle edges have been lifted up by a harsh shampoo or hard water, or if your hair tends to "fly-away" when it's dry or becomes "frizzy" when it's wet, then a creme rinse may solve your problems.

The "creme" effect is actually only a cosmetic trick to enhance the image of a product that is supposed to cream or soften hair. The conditioning agent—a chemical "surfactant" that sticks to and coats the hair—isn't "creamy" at all but rather dissolves into a clear solution.

When the conditioning agent fixes to the hair's surface, it flattens the cuticle returning natural sheen and actually increases refractive properties, thereby *adding* sheen. Moreover, it effectively neutralizes any static electric changes on the hair's surface, reducing any tendency for fly-away.

Creme rinses are always formulated as acids to help neutralize alkaline cleansers and further aid in returning the cuticle to its natural state.

The popular commercial products tend to be oriented to a female market.

> Agree creme rinse
> Breck creme rinse
> Lemon Up creme rinse
> Tame creme rinse

"Instant" Conditioners

This is the most commonly used type of conditioner. The products are actually creme rinses with added "body builders." They do exactly what the creme rinses do—but perhaps a little better.

The term "instant" refers to the fact that they—like creme rinses—are left on the hair for about a minute before being rinsed away. Like creme rinses, they are always acidic, are anti-static, and contain a conditioning surfactant agent.

The added body builders commonly include oils, fats, waxes, esters, vitamins and proteins. They provide added lubrication for the hair which gains more luster and smoothness. Proteins may further enhance this effect by penetrating into the hair shaft to build "body" from within. This may be especially useful when dealing with damaged, fine or thinned-out hair.

In addition to being sold as instant conditioners, they may be called a "creme rinse and conditioner" or a "balsam conditioner." Balsam conditioners, by the way, do not usually contain balsams. The term does not refer to the chemical balsams obtained from trees and shrubs, but rather, is used in a literal sense to imply "smoothness" and "gentleness." The fragrance of most products suitable for use by either sex:

Alberto Balsam
Revlon Flex Balsam & Protein (regular or extra body)
Wella Balsam (regular or extra body)

Based on fragrance, for women only:
Clairol Short & Sassy, or Long & Silky
Earth Born (in various fruit flavors)

For men only:
Dep for Men

"Deep Down" Conditioners

These products are essentially like the preceding type, only more so. Since damaged hair accepts conditioning agents and body builders more readily than normal hair, deep down conditioners are provided with more of these substances.

They will penetrate and coat the hair, filling in surface cracks and increasing luster. They're meant for "problem hair" that is either naturally dry or brittle or made that way through bleaching, dyeing, straightening or perming. They are usually left on the hair for at least five minutes before being rinsed out.

The products are usually marketed for women.
Breck Satin creme conditioner
Clairol Condition
Revlon Flex Balsam & Protein
Wella Kolestral
Alberto Hot Oil Treatment is used before shampooing. This type of treatment has been used in beauty parlors for lubricating a dry scalp. For deep down conditioning of hair, I think that the other products in this group are simpler to use and just as effective.

Setting Lotion Conditioners

These—and the following group—are applied after shampooing and are not rinsed out. Like hair dressings and sprays, they are used primarily to promote hair manageability.

Their essential ingredients are resins—either natural compounds such as shellac or, more likely, vinyl "polymers" (chemicals made up of smaller units numbering in the millions).

Resins coat hair, fixing it in place. Since they tend to dry and crack, they are "softened" by special additives. Once softened, they will hold the hair, yet keep it manageable.

To enhance their conditioning capabilities, the same kind of agents found in instant and deep down conditioners are added, hence the name setting lotion *conditioner.*

These products are formulated in lotion or gel form and are generally marketed for women. A few are suitable for men who need to add body and increase manageability of their hair.

Alberto VO5 Hair Setting Gel or Lotion
Breck Basic Conditioner
Dep balsam styling gel
Dippity-Do (line includes conditioning gels)
Kindness (Clairol)
L'Oréal Naturally Free setting lotion
Power Pal (Clairol)
Protein 21 conditioner (for men also)
Protein 29 hair groom spray (marketed for men)
Salon Finish (Breck) (for men also)
Thicket (for men also)
Wella Care Do (for men also)
Wellaflex setting lotion

Hair Sprays

I've included this group because they are usually formulated like setting lotion conditioners but *without* conditioners or body builders. They contain resins that are not overly "softened" in order to retain a better hold and coat the hair with a relatively inelastic film.

They have replaced the drying alcoholic lotions and greasy pomades of a quarter century ago as the modern way for fixing hair in place once it has been "set."

People often ask if inhalation of hair sprays can damage lungs. The particles that make up the spray mist are actually too large to penetrate deep enough into our lungs to create any damage. Because most hair sprays are perfumed, they should be used in well-ventilated areas, not to avoid lung irritation but to reduce nasal discomfort.

Most hair sprays marketed today work as well as competing brands and are formulated for either men or women by variations in fragrance. Their resin concentration—or "holding power"—varies as well as their packaging into aerosol or non-aerosol containers. Gel hair dressings, usually favored by men, are actually similar products but are packaged in tubes.

You might require one or several kinds of conditioners to properly groom your hair. While they cannot really repair damages, they can change the physical properties of hair in order to make it look and feel better.

The need for conditioning may vary with the climate, being more helpful when hair is dried by lower winter humidity or excessive summer sun, the kind of shampoo you use, the frequency of shampooing, and the inherent manageability of your hair.

10

Changing the Shape and Color of Hair

SINCE "UNISEX" STYLING HAS become so commonplace, any discussion about waving, straightening or coloring hair need no longer be reserved "for women only." Today, both sexes benefit from most—if not all—of these cosmetic applications.

For each group, I'll again list several of the more popular commercial products. If none of these listed are available, chances are your druggist, beautician or barber will have other products that are equally good.

CHANGING THE SHAPE OF HAIR

Permanent Waving

Although electric curlers are back with us again, most permanent waving is performed by protein-splitting agents called thioglycolates. They were introduced in the '40's as the "cold wave" and are still popular today.

The difference between a cold wave and a "body wave" is simply the size of the rod used to set the hair. The body wave employs a larger rod to create a wave with less curl.

After hair is curled or "set" into position, a thioglycolate lotion is applied to break the protein bonds that form the chemical "skeleton" of hair. This destructive process is called a "reduction."

Since thioglycolates also happen to be the active ingredients of some depilatories, cold wave perming must be performed carefully to avoid hair breakage. Perming of wiry, brittle or damaged hair should probably not be attempted because breakage is likely.

Following the reduction step, a peroxide solution is applied to neutralize the waving reaction and re-form the protein bonds, which now hold the hair in its new shape. This rejuvenation process is called an "oxidation."

Today, the market for home cold waving products has "contracted," because the new styles favor shorter hair that is usually worn straight or natural. Additionally, many cosmetic firms have chosen to avail these products for professional use only because of safety factors.

Some of the home perming products include:
Extra Body Perm kit (L'Oréal)
Fast Home Permanent Kit (Rexall)
Full Body (L'Oréal)
Lilt (Proctor & Gamble)
Ogilvie (Tussy)
Quick (Richard Hudnut)
Toni (Gillette)

Temporary Waving

A "wave set" will curl or wave hair temporarily—shampooing will return the hair to its former shape.

The simplest way to accomplish this is to wet the hair and fix it in place with or without rollers and blow it dry. To increase the holding action, a setting gel, lotion, cream or spray may be applied before drying.

Straightening Hair

The older methods of straightening hair employed hot irons combined with oils to distribute the heat or simple "pressing" of hair with an electric iron. Not only did hair breakage and scalp irritation occur frequently, scarring and permanent hair loss could result, especially when heat-conducting oils were used.

Three types of chemical "relaxers" have now essentially replaced heat straightening methods. While they work quickly and efficiently, they too are capable of creating skin and hair damage. The incidence of irritating reactions has been reported as high as 8%.

Not only must they be used carefully, they should not be expected to accomplish too much. For example, if your hair is kinky, settle for "straighter" hair with a wave in it. If your hair is dyed or bleached, don't attempt to straighten it more than once every four to six months. Improper applications may provide you with plenty of straight hair—everywhere but on your scalp!

Alkali Straighteners

Most chemical straighteners used in this country today are in this group. They work the fastest—in about five to ten minutes—but they also are the most caustic. While they are primarily used professionally, some alkali products (containing sodium hydroxide) are available for home use.

Ever Perm (Helene Curtis)
Hair Strate (Summit Laboratories)
Realistic Permanent Creme Hair Relaxer (Revlon)
Ultra Sheen (Johnson Products Co.)

Thioglycolate Straighteners

Often referred to as "reverse permanent waves," they are most used professionally. They work in about ten to fifteen minutes and must be neutralized with an oxidizer as in the cold waving process. While they are safer than alkali straighteners, they may not be quite as effective. Several are sold for home use.

Curls Away (Richard Hudnut)
Perma Strate (Perma Strate Co.)
Set Me Straight (Rexall)
Smooth Away (Helene Curtis)
Straight Set (Max Factor)

Bisulfite Straighteners

These agents represent the newest group of "curl relaxers." They are more effective than the thioglycolates and are safer and almost as effective as the alkalies. They are left on the hair for about fifteen minutes and must be neutralized. While used professionally, they also have the largest share of the "home market."

Charles Antell Curl Relaxing Formula (Charles Antell)
Curl Free (Prom Cosmetics—Gillette)
Curlaxer (Posner)
U.N.C.U.R.L. (Clairol)

CHANGING THE COLOR OF HAIR

Hair coloring changes hair shades, which may be thought of as variations of the color brown.

The highlights of this color differentiate *hues*. Hues are

classified as "drab" (blue), "ash" (green), "warm" (red), or "golden" (yellow).

While most products display color charts demonstrating their shades, the final result will be influenced by your natural color. Before applying any hair color, you should perform a "strand test." By coloring one or several strands of hair, you can learn how to use the product properly while evaluating your new hair shade.

Hair color may be altered on a *permanent*, *semi-permanent* or *temporary* basis.

Permanent Hair Coloring

Vegetable dyes were first used 4,000 years ago. The leaves of the henna plant probably reddened Cleopatra's hair; but by the early part of this century, this dye lost favor because it usually produced an unnatural orange-red color.

Today, it has been reborn as a "natural hair treatment." Red henna (from the leaves), black henna (from the roots), and neutral henna (from the stem) are being used to create subtle color changes, although the dye tends to wear off after several months, and as conditioning agents, to coat hair promoting thickness and shine.

Henna, while quite safe for hair, is tricky to work with and probably should only be used professionally. Unfortunately, it creates an artificial looking hair color.

Metallic dyes, usually lead or silver, coat hair and react with its protein to leave the permanent color of the particular metal used.

These are the dyes that have become popular with men who want to "cover the gray" slowly over a period of weeks.

They are safe and easy to use, combed in daily until the hair darkens sufficiently. Unfortunately, they may produce an unnatural dyed look and hair brittleness.

Grecian Formula 16 (Combe)
Lady Grecian Formula (Combe)
RD for Men (LT Industries)
Youthair (Majestic Drug Co.)

Tints are now the most commonly used permanent dyes. They start out as colorless chemicals—usually combinations of phenol compounds and other agents—that take on color when peroxide is added to the mix just before being rubbed into the hair.

They're also called "oxidation" dyes, because they must be oxidized (by peroxide) to couple the colorless intermediate chemicals.

Within the past ten years, tints have become extremely sophisticated cosmetic preparations that are now quite safe for home use, if used properly. Up to ten different chemicals, each with its own peroxide oxidizer, plus some pre-formed dyes may combine to produce a given shade. The peroxide is added to the preparation by the user immediately before use. The commercial products most often are sold in lotion, aerosol or shampoo form.

The two main advantages of these oxidation dyes are the variety of *lasting natural shades* that are available and their ability to *lighten* hair slightly (because of the added peroxide) as well as darken it. Colorists call this a "single process," because only one step is necessary to change hair color.

While the incidence of allergic reactions are quite low with these dyes, the potential for skin eruptions, consisting of redness, swelling and itching on the scalp and face does exist. The package insert will state this fact and provide instructions for patch testing, which should be performed prior to *each* usage.

Other peroxide products such as cold wave preparations should not be used over these dyes since the chances for hair discoloration and breakage are quite great. If you perm or straighten your hair, do it *before* you color it.

There are too many commerical products available to list here. Tints can be identified by a warning about skin reactions, patch test instructions, a suggestion to re-apply no sooner than every three to four weeks, and a statement that the dye provides a permanent color that cannot be shampooed out.

Bleaches are essentially hydrogen peroxide combined with a variety of stabilizers to prevent its decomposition and accelerators to improve its efficiency. This method of lightening hair color is also called "stripping," "blonding," or "lifting."

The oxidation of hair with peroxide is performed as the first step to achieve the desired lighter tone. Since the hair often turns the wrong shade of yellow, a second "toning" step follows. A hair *toner* is simply a tint used to create an attractive shade in bleached hair.

This two-step procedure, or "double process," can achieve drastic color change. The simpler, safer and now more popular single process required by tints can lighten hair, but only with a double process can you go from black to blond.

Again, too many products are available for listing. In general, bleaches will usually have the words "Lightener," "Blonde" or "Bleach" to identify them, while toners are usually referred to as such. They may be sold as double process kits (including kits for frosting and tipping) or sold separately as bleaches and toners.

Allergic reactions may occur with bleaches as well as toners. Some of the chemical accelerators are known allergens that have produced reactions ranging from mild hay fever to severe respiratory distress requiring hospitalization. Additionally, the alkalinity of the bleaching solution may produce chemical skin burns. Patch tests, unfortunately, are not predictive.

Caution should be exercised with regard to trying to accomplish too much lightening of darker hair too often. Overbleached hair is dry, dull and brittle. While conditioners may help, often the only restorative "treatment" is simply to let the new hair grow in and try to accomplish less lightening the next time.

Semi-Permanent Hair Coloring

These dyes were originally borrowed from the textile industry. They were usually shampooed into the hair and left in place for about a half hour to be oxidized slowly by the air. Today, most cosmetic companies have developed special non-oxidizing dyes that simply diffuse into the hair.

These dyes are called "semi-permanent," because while they penetrate the hair shaft, they tend to wash out after five or six shampoos.

Properly used, they can change shades within a narrow range of the individual's natural color. Although the dyes vary from blond to black, they can never *lighten* hair because they do not contain peroxide.

Because they are safe and simple to use, they have become quite popular and appear to be replacing many permanent dyes as color additives.

Like tints, semi-permanent dyes may (rarely) produce allergic reactions and should be patch tested prior to use. The package label will state that no mixing is required and that the color should be expected to last through four or five shampoos.

Several popular products for home use include:
Color 'n' Tone (Nestlé-Le Mur)
Happiness (Clairol)
Loving Care (Clairol)
Silk and Silver (Clairol)
Touch of Silver (L'Oréal)

Temporary Hair Coloring

Temporary dyes coat the surface of the hair with a color that can be washed out after one shampoo. They are usually quite safe to use and no longer rub off easily when the hair is accidentally moistened.

They are formulated into color rinses, sets and shampoos, and are used mostly in soft light shades to create highlights and add sheen to gray or white hair.

Temporary hair colors available as rinses include:

Instant Come Alive Gray (Clairol)
Nestle Protein Colorinse (Nestlé-Le Mur)
Noreen Color Hair Rinse (Noreen)
Picture Perfect Instant Color Rinse (Clairol)

11

Styling Hair

FOR ALMOST AS LONG A man has had scalp hair and a useful instrument with which to cut it, custom has dictated that it be styled in a particular fashion. We are now living in an era in which styling methods have not only become more interesting but more sensible and easy to manage by oneself.

We now possess the most sophisticated and practical cosmetic products with which to clean, condition, alter shape and color, and fix hair in place. Anyone should be able to style his or her hair in a manner that will enhance its natural beauty without "coiffuring" it into an artificial canopy.

To achieve a comfortable and attractive hairstyle, you will certainly require professional help. But to succeed, you should rid yourself of the habit of having a barber or beautician cut and set your hair as if it were a museum piece to be viewed and not handled between visits.

The Hair Stylist

The term "stylist," unlike "barber" or "beautician," suggests the promise that our hair, whether or not we're satisfied with it, will somehow be made to look better through his or her expertise.

This expectation, however, is not always fulfilled. Styling hair properly demands more than technical skills—it requires an artistic flair. You may have to shop around for the right stylist and often be willing to pay a higher premium to achieve a satisfactory hairdo.

Your Hair Style

While you should avoid using a stylist who "specializes" in a particular hairdo that he duplicates on the head of all his customers, you should similarly avoid trying to make your hair into something it isn't, simply because the style is popular.

The quantity and texture of your hair will usually dictate the kind of style that best suits it.

Your age, height, weight and facial contours need also be considered.

Even your self-image should be considered when accepting or rejecting various styles.

There really aren't any fixed rules to follow anymore. Many tall young women often wear short hair quite well, while many older men manage to look quite proper with longer collar-length hair.

The Haircut

Most stylists agree that the way in which hair is cut is the key to a correct hairstyle. Until it grows out, your hair should be "programmed" by the stylist's scissors to maintain its form even after it's been shampooed.

The scissors is the essential tool of the craft. Used properly, it creates the least hair damage. By cutting straight across the ends of the hair, the remaining shaft is not disturbed and its natural "body" remains intact. On the other hand, when hair is razor cut, it tends to lie flat because the ends become tapered by the diagonal slicing action of that instrument. In addition to loss of "body," razor cutting may tear apart the cuticle of the hair creating dullness and tangling.

By cutting a group of hairs in equal lengths but varying the lengths of adjacent groups, a "layered" effect is achieved which also contributes to "body." Layered cutting is especially helpful to people possessing poor hair density. *Short* layered hair has fullness. Trying to make up in length what you lack in density is usually self-defeating because longer hair—while there is certainly more of it—tends to flatten and lie limp under its own weight, that is, it has no "body."

Having your hair cut regularly also solves the problem of how to deal with dull "weathered" and split ends—they're simply removed.

Styling Tricks for Thinned Hair

Aside from wearing your hair shorter and having it "layered" properly, there are other useful ways to achieve the look of density.

Changing the shape of your hair from straight to wavy or curly will "hide the scalp" more effectively.

Lightening your hair color can lessen the contrast between hair and scalp, enhancing, at least, the illusion of density.

Moving the part further over to one side of your scalp and "sweeping" hair across the thinned area may cover it more effectively.

Combing hair forward can hide a recessed hairline. The "Caesar" cut for men and the use of bangs for women accomplishes this kind of benign deception.

Frequent shampooing helps by removing the excess oil that contributes to matting of hair. Freshly washed hair always has more body.

Conditioning properly can thicken individual hairs by coating them to add fullness to fine or thinned hair.

Blow drying or hot combing encourages "controlled fly-away" (and more "body") by removing the water that acts as a conductor of the weak electric charges that attract and mat individual hairs to their neighbors.

When styling your thinned hair, avoid over-teasing, lowering the part too close to one ear, sweeping hair forward from the nape of the neck, or allowing sideburns to grow down to the jawline. These "tricks" seem not to conceal your problems, but rather draw attention to them.

Useful Styling Methods for Setting Hair

After your hair has been shampooed, you will probably "set" it into place with either a comb, brush or by a more elaborate method. While women tend to use more accessories for setting hair, both sexes today share many aids, such as hair blowers and dressings.

The important concept to be remembered is that your hair needn't appear the same every day. If it has been cut, shampooed and conditioned properly, it may look slightly different if you re-style it yourself, but it can certainly look good and feel more comfortable because it's clean.

The simplest way to set hair is the method most men and women use—the "place set." Damp hair is simply combed or brushed into place and, as it's dried naturally or with the aid of a blower or hot comb, it "sets" into place.

A "blow-dry" set is essentially the same process. The hair is simply manipulated more into its new position by a brush while it is dried with a mechanical blower.

Using setting lotion conditioners, hair gels or dressings, wire mesh or plastic or electric rollers, bobby pins, clips or elastic bands can increase the complexity of a set. Most of these measures are more likely to be used by women who, if they are proficient enough, may even recreate the same hairdo that they had when they left their beauty parlors.

Styling Methods to Avoid

Along with the aforementioned warnings against over-bleaching, over-dyeing, over-straightening, over-perming and razor cutting, several other methods should either be avoided or used only with extreme caution.

Most stylists oppose thinning out hair because it tends to produce damaged hairs of unequal lengths, thereby negating the methods used to create body.

Stiff nylon brushes and fine-toothed combs may damage hair especially if it's kinky or wet. Whatever grooming devices you choose, you should keep them clean, but don't worry about "sterilizing" them, because scalp and hair infections are fairly uncommon.

Backcombing (teasing) hair may add "lift" when used judiciously, but more often this styling method creates premature breakage and split ends by literally stripping off the cuticle from its shaft.

Hot air dryers should be kept at least six inches from the hair and always moving in order to avoid singeing the hair and breaking it.

The use of hair sprays is often frowned upon by stylists, but they certainly can be helpful. Since sprays "weld" adjacent hairs together at their cross-over points, they are applied as the final step in the grooming process. Re-brushing tends to peel them off the hairs creating "false dandruff."

Once you understand the kinds of cleansing, grooming and styling aids available, you should be able—with minimal effort—to make the most of what you have.

There are plenty of fine products available for you to use. While the language of the stylist, cosmetologist and advertising person may sometimes confuse you (and me), the classification of commercial aids is actually fairly simple.

Try to clean your hair and scalp often.

If necessary, find the kind of conditioner that suits your particular hair texture and environment.

If desired, change your hair shape or color on a permanent or temporary basis.

Certainly have your hair cut properly and "set" it to your taste.

It is really quite easy to do.

Be yourself and enjoy your hair!

REPLACING IT IF IT'S GONE

IV

The Cosmetic Replacement of Hair

JULIUS CAESAR MAY have started it all.

Since he was alleged to have received a special dispensation from the Roman Senate to cover his balding head with a crown, people have searched for ways less regal to conceal their barren scalps. Over the past two thousand years, hairpieces, in one form or another, have been the most popular cosmetic accessory used for this purpose.

Physical appeal has always assumed an important role in an individual's ability to achieve success. Today, our society has transformed this concept into a kind of youth-worship. Without youth and beauty, one might become socially—and perhaps even economically—handicapped.

No matter how we cut it, an attractive crop of scalp hair contributes significantly to our concept of a youthful appearance. Since our self-image develops during our younger "hairier" years, it is no wonder that so many try so hard to display a full head of hair even if it must be gained artificially.

Because a hairpiece is an easily removable appliance, it may restrict its wearer's participation in certain activities. For some people this lack of permanence creates a sense of insecurity. To relieve this anxiety—or perhaps to fuel it—a mini-industry hawking "permanent" hairpieces has mushroomed over the past few years.

In this section, I'll discuss the various kinds of removable hairpieces available today and the two methods that are currently popular for fixing extra hair "permanently" to the scalp.

12. HAIRPIECES
13. HAIR WEAVING
14. HAIR IMPLANTING

12

Hairpieces

THE ANCIENT EGYPTIANS were the first group of people to cover their heads with something other than their own hair. The term *head*piece, however, would best describe the kind of appliance they chose to wear.

Perhaps, because they eschewed hair as something barbaric, they shaved their heads and designed their headpieces to suggest—but not simulate—scalp hair. This affectation was strictly upper class. In fact, the headpiece identified its wearer as an important person.

During the sixteenth and seventeenth centuries, intricate headpieces containing human and animal hair were created. By the eighteenth century, they became immensely popular not only for covering "noble" heads but for most people who could afford them, including liveried servants. People wearing wigs made no attempt to conceal the fact that they weren't displaying their own hair. Besides, the size, density and variation in color of most hairpieces became so ridiculously extravagant, that they left no doubt about their artificial nature.

The hairpiece was a fashion the early settlers brought to this country. Wigs remained in vogue from our colonial period until the early nineteenth century. They gradually became more realistic as the style was to use them to fill out—not cover—one's own hair. Thereafter, their role was reduced to that of a theatrical prop. By the mid-twentieth century, they reappeared—but primarily for hiding baldness.

The machine age completely democratized the hairpiece. A wig or toupee can now be produced so inexpensively that anybody can afford one—or several—to either cover baldness or conveniently change a hairstyle.

A "*Piece*" for Every Need

There's one for most styling needs.

For the man or woman desiring to cover a balding scalp or change a hairstyle, the full hairpiece, or *wig* does it easily. The pre-styled hair is usually attached to an elastic base so that the wig can be fitted to the head and worn like a cap.

Hairpieces that cover only part of the head are attached by either adhesive to a bald scalp or tied or clipped to underlying hair.

A bald man wears a *toupee* that partially covers the scalp and blends into his side and rear fringe of hair.

Women's partial hairpieces are defined by their size and length of hair. A *wiglet* covers part of the scalp with short hair. If the wiglet provides more coverage, it's called a *cascade* . A *fall* does the same thing but with longer hair. A *switch* is a kind of narrow fall. When several switches are braided or twisted together at the back of the head, they form a *chignon.*

The Hair That Never Grows

It may be natural or synthetic.

Sheep, yaks and Angora goats donate their fleece for wigs that are used for theatrical purposes. The most desirable hair used for hairpieces is sheared from human scalps. Traditionally, the choicest—and most expensive—hair comes from Northern Europe because it is finely textured and available in a variety of colors. Oriental hair, being less expensive, is now quite popular, but it tends to be coarser and limited to darker colors.

When hair is used in its natural state, it's referred to as "raw." "Processed" means that the hair has been either dyed, bleached and/or reshaped.

Because it never grows, the hair on a piece cannot be altered or "processed" repeatedly, or it will break. It must, however, be cleaned and conditioned regularly to keep it looking attractive.

Synthetic or man-made hair, formed from modified acrylic ("modacrylic") fiber such as Dynel®, Kanekalon® and Elura®, has become the staple of the stretch wig industry.

These synthetic fibers have great mass-market appeal because they're cheaper than—and remarkably similar to—human hair. Moreover, they don't mat or tangle, stay cleaner and hold their shape and color better than real hair. Stretch wigs containing synthetic hair are usually produced in the Far East. In 1976, we imported 15 million of them!

What You Can't See Really Matters

The kind and quantity of hair used in a piece, the way it matches the person's own hair and the mixing of colors to achieve subtle changes in the tone or "salt-and-pepper" effects, all add to the attractiveness—and cost—of any hairpiece.

How this hair is attached to its base, however, is equally critical for achieving a more natural effect.

The best bases are handmade. They're called "ventilated" because they're made from lightweight materials that allow air to reach the scalp, such as nylon, silk, cotton net and gauze. Because they're hand tied, individual hairs can be spaced properly to create a more natural appearance.

Additional refinements include elastic skin-like materials incorporated into the base—usually around the part—to simulate scalp and lace fronts which are glued to the forehead to create an "invisible" hairline—as long as the forehead remains free of natural oils and perspiration.

Machine-made hairpieces are called "wefted" because hairs are attached to the base in groups—or wefts—rather than singly. While the bases used for these hairpieces are inexpensive, they tend to be bulkier and less comfortable than hand-tied bases. For example, the ready-to-wear stretch wigs employ elastic bases, warmer than nylon or gauze but flexible enough to slip on over a full head of hair.

The Advantages of Wearing a Hairpiece

For people with plenty of hair but the wrong hairstyle, a full stretch wig may permit them to instantly change their coiffure. While less popular than they were several years ago, these wigs can still ease the bondage of women to their beauty parlors, especially when time or distance makes a visit impractical.

For women desiring to "dress up" their hairdos, the various kinds of partial hairpieces are especially helpful.

For any kind of baldness, a partial or full hairpiece is still the most popular accessory used to replace lost hair.

The most significant advantage of a hairpiece is that it is safe to use and easy to put on and remove. Despite some old wives' tales, wigs and toupees do not encourage hair loss or cultivate scalp infections provided that they're attached properly, removed nightly and kept clean along with their owners' own hair and scalp.

The Disadvantages of Wearing a Hairpiece

Toupees and wigs cover large scalp areas. While a scalp

doesn't "breathe," it does perspire. By occluding the scalp, a piece may make it warm and uncomfortable.

If a hairpiece is worn regularly, it should be cleaned almost weekly—and professionally. Purchasing a piece, owning a spare, maintaining both and replacing them every few years may involve cost factors that become a disadvantage.

Activities such as swimming are usually difficult—or impossible—to manage while wearing a hairpiece.

A natural looking irregular hairline is impossible to duplicate without creating special "invisible" gauze-like meshes that must be glued to the forehead and become only too visible after several hours of wear.

Many pieces must be constructed of a mix of about 40% human and 60% synthetic hair, because while human hair provides natural color and texture, it wears out faster than its synthetic counterparts.

The feeling that no matter how good it looks, you're still wearing something atop your head that isn't your own hair turns off many potential customers.

Finally, the fact that you can't wear it constantly bothers many people. While people wearing eyeglasses or false teeth accept this kind of limitation, enough dissatisfied toupee wearers exist to have created a large market for "permanent" hairpieces. The methods used to achieve permanence will be described in the following two chapters.

13

Hair Weaving

A "NON-SURGICAL METHOD for achieving permanent hair" is the way you'll read about it.

The process is usually promoted by advertisements that are often quite enticing. Look for photographs of neatly coiffured famous athletes, people vigorously lathering their weaves in a shower, or men effortlessly swimming beside attractive long-haired (but unweaved) women.

Hair weaving originated with Black people more than a century ago. One could say that they were the first to search for a way to enrich their "roots." Today, weaves have achieved a wider popularity, but they seem to be losing ground to the newer implanting processes (see chapter 14).

Both weaving and implanting services are usually offered by "*replace*-your-hair clinics" that may or may not be part of a "*save-* your-hair" facility (see chapter 4). Many of these "clinics" have now begun to perform hair transplantation, a procedure that properly belongs in a physician's office or hospital.

While I cannot personally endorse these clinics or the weaving process, I would encourage anyone choosing a weave to carefully check out the organization performing this service with your local Better Business Bureau. Furthermore, I would strongly advise anyone contemplating hair weaving to meet people who have been wearing one for a while, rather than making a decision based only upon promotional material.

What Is a Hair Weave?

Weaving hair really means braiding it—tightly—so that a toupee or smaller weft can be attached "permanently." All you require is enough hair remaining on your scalp to serve as an anchor for a hairpiece.

The braids are usually formed from the thicker hair found on the sides and back of the scalp. A semicircular ridge is created that holds a toupee firmly in place (figure 6).

If enough hair is still growing on the top of the scalp, it can be twisted into smaller braids to anchor individual wefts. This type of weave permits better aeration and easier cleansing of the scalp.

What Is a Hair Fusion?

A "fusion," "bonding," or "linking" is exactly like a weave

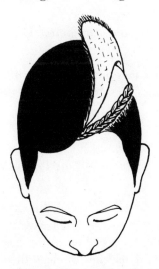

Figure 6. HAIR WEAVE: **The hair remaining on the sides of the scalp is tightly braided. The braids serve as an "anchor" to which a toupee is attached.**

except that the toupee or wefts are *glued*, instead of tied, onto the braided hair. This so-called "chemical bond" is water-insoluble and, unfortunately, quite caustic. Frequent hair breakage has limited the usefulness of this method.

Do Weaves and Fusions Require Special Care?

While weaved or fused hair does not grow, it still requires regular care and maintenance to keep it looking acceptable. Like any hair accessory that is worn regularly, it may wear out after months or years.

The scalp hair, used to anchor the weave, naturally continues to grow. As it grows, the attached hair starts to ride above the scalp. The weave or fusion must be re-anchored frequently—as often as every three weeks.

Do Weaves or Fusions Look Any Better Than Removable Hairpieces?

Aside from the convenience of wearing them to bed or under water, they offer no significant cosmetic advantage over a toupee or a smaller "partial" hairpiece.

What Are the Disadvantages of This Type of Hair Replacement?

Since most people who choose this type of replacement have too little hair left to anchor smaller wefts, they simply wind up with a toupee tightly attached to the hair of the sides and back of their scalps. This kind of close fit does not make for proper hygiene. Scalp scales, dirt and left-over shampoo tend to accumulate within the braids forming a soggy residue that may irritate the scalp. Even when wefts are used, the braided areas are difficult to cleanse. Additionally, the attached hair—like any hair accessory—may not hold up well under the kind of shampooing we normally use for our hair and scalps.

The frequent rebraiding sessions, aside from consuming both time and money, leave the scalp feeling uncomfortable because a weave is usually tightly applied. By the time it loosens and becomes comfortable, it may have lifted enough to require rebraiding.

A weave or fusion, like any artificial hair accessory, requires careful daily maintenance. Whether toupeed, wefted or fused, the hair must be styled well or it will look ridiculous.

The most distressing disadvantage of weaving or fusing concerns the tension placed upon the anchoring scalp hair. Chronic tension placed upon scalp hair usually creates accelerated shedding. This hair loss is similar to that experienced by ponytail wearers—and it often is *irreversible*.

I imagine that most people wear a hairpiece to try to forget that they're bald—at least while it's on. The person wearing a toupee or wig accomplishes this until it's removed at bedtime. The person wearing a hairweave or fusion postpones this "letdown" at least until it has to be reset. He or she is, however, only *exchanging* one incovenience for another, while often forfeiting a clean scalp and perhaps sacrificing a great deal of the treasured remaining hair.

14

Hair Implanting

HAIR IMPLANTING HAS BEEN hailed—by its promoters—as the "ultimate permanent hair replacement" and a "miraculous surgical process not involving transplants."

Also known less pretentiously as "medical" or "suture" implants, it has become the principal method for fixing a hairpiece securely to the scalp. Unfortunately, its popularity has aroused the avaricious instincts of many fly-by-night hair-replacement clinic operators who, in the wake of their departure, have left behind a large array of dissatisfied customers.

Even under ideal circumstances, implants are usually far from permanent, only quasi-medical and in no way should be confused with transplants to which they share a resemblance in name only.

What Is an Implant?

Implants are stitches—made from either stainless steel or nylon-type materials—that are sewn into the scalp and tied into rings. Like the weave hair braids, the knotted stitches act as anchors, holding a toupee or several wefts against the barren scalp.

If the implants secure a toupee, only two or perhaps a half-dozen stitches are needed.

If the implants anchor many smaller wefts of hair, more than a dozen stitches must be sewn into the scalp. Figure 7 illustrates a "double ring" pattern of implants with a single weft fixed in place.

Doesn't This Procedure Require a Physician's Participation?

Yes. Only someone possessing a medical license can inject a local anesthetic and sew stitches into the scalp.

A physician must be hired by an implant clinic to perform this service. While he may suture the scalp in his own office, everything else—the promotions, payments, hairpiece design and follow-up care —is usually assumed by the clinic operators, without any medical supervision.

In general, the medical profession does not condone implanting, because the difficulties encountered with this procedure far outweigh any of the expected benefits.

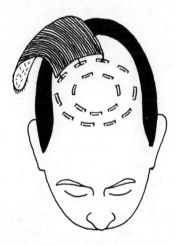

Figure 7. HAIR IMPLANT: Stitches are sewn into the scalp. In this illustration, three stitches serve as "anchors" for a weft of hair.
If wefts are used, many stitches must be sewn. If a toupee is worn, fewer stitches are used but the tension on each is greater.

Why Has Implanting Become More Popular Than Weaving?

The promise that the attached hairpiece will somehow remain "permanently" fixed to the scalp appears more possible with an implant than a weave. Since the hair accessory is not anchored to anything that can grow away from the scalp, there is no need for the frequent rebraidings characteristic of weaves.

Furthermore, since the candidate need not contribute any of his or her own hair, even total baldness isn't an excuse for foregoing an implant.

But aside from these two factors, the cosmetic result delivered by this process is no better than that offered by a weave or a removable wig or toupee.

What Are the Disadvantages of Implants?

Many of the disadvantages associated with weaves and taped-on hairpieces apply to implants. Implants, however, introduce one factor that creates problems far greater than that seen with other hair replacement methods. The problems generated by sewing—and leaving—stitches in the scalp may become overwhelming, despite claims to the contrary.

The major difficulty with retained stitches is that they create permanent tunnels in the scalp which may foster bacterial growth. When bacteria grow unchecked, infections follow. I have treated several people who required large doses of antibiotics for their implant-induced scalp infections. Because the scalp's rich blood supply connects to the brain via the veins of the face, the potential for a brain infection is very real—enough to frighten me away from recommending this process.

A problem that is slow to develop but almost certain to occur involves scarring. No matter how "inert" implant stitches are claimed to be, they are always treated by the scalp as foreign irritants. While it is true that these stitches are the same type used to repair a damaged heart, they leave scars—but only in the scalp will they feel uncomfortable.

When the scars produce discomfort—as they often do—the stitches must be removed and new ones sewn into other areas of the scalp. Over the years, the top of the head may become a patchwork quilt of scars.

There are several minor difficulties that may become quite disconcerting.

Freshly implanted stitches, like a newly tightened weave, usually hurt. Many people have said that it takes months to accommodate to the pain.

Scalp hygiene may be compromised, especially if the implants are anchoring a close-fitting toupee. While individual wefts may minimize this difficulty, the extra sutures required may create their own problems.

The somewhat tenuous attachment of the hairpiece to the anchoring sutures has resulted in yet another type of minor disaster. Scalp lacerations have been reported in people who accidentally—or purposely—had their hairpieces pulled out.

Can Implanting Be Performed Without Stitches?

Recently, a surgical procedure known as "tunnel grafting" has been developed that is *not* available in implant clinics.

A one-by-three-inch rectangle of skin is removed from behind each ear. The two pieces are immediately grafted to the front and back of the scalp to form two loops that serve as anchors for a toupee.

While the operation is fairly simple to perform, extreme care must be taken to insure proper graft acceptance and healing.

Although this method avoids the pitfalls of implanted stitches, it still retains two of the problems common to any kind of artificial anchoring device.

Since only two loops are available to fix a hairpiece, only a toupee can be worn. A toupee held down at only two points can still lift off the scalp.

The skin loops are as vulnerable to injury as suture loops. Scalp lacerations resulting from forcible removable of the toupee have occurred.

I remember asking one of my patients why he exchanged his removable toupee for an implant. He said that he couldn't face the embarrassment of having his toupee pop off during a moment of passion with his girlfriend. I wondered about the embarrassment he might feel if she ever ran her hand through his wefted hair and caught a finger in one of the suture loops!

Once again, the choice of an implant over a taped-on hairpiece really amounts to exchanging one set of inconveniences for another. The removable wig or toupee achieves the same basic cosmetic effect, and recently developed taping adhesives keep most toupees tightly bonded to the scalp. Moreover, if you tire of wearing your hairpiece, you can easily discard it without having compromised your remaining hair or scalp.

V

The Surgical Replacement of Hair

THERE ARE THREE reasonable approaches for dealing with your baldness—either ignore it, wear a good hairpiece, or have a hair transplant.

Since the discovery, made nearly twenty years ago, that surgery could correct baldness permanently, approximately a million people—both men and women—have undergone transplants. Most significantly, at least half this number have been treated in only the past half decade.

While this surge in transplant popularity is quite impressive, it has not been accompanied by a lessening of the confusion and misunderstandings among many potential candidates. Most information dealing with this topic has been provided by a "show-and-tell" kind of television and magazine coverage. While this type of reporting certainly generates interest in the procedure, it does not usually offer meaningful explanations of what it's really all about.

In this section, I'll discuss the typical questions asked by people who are considering a hair transplant. The following chapters should answer most of the questions you'd ever care to ask about this procedure:

15. CHOOSING THE RIGHT DOCTOR
16. WHAT COMMON BALDNESS IS REALLY ABOUT
17. HOW HAIR IS TRANSPLANTED

15

Choosing the Right Doctor

IF YOU SUDDENLY "doubled-up" from a sharp knife-like pain in
your right lower abdomen and thought you had appendicitis,
would you reach for your daily newspaper to find an ad for an
"appendectomy clinic?"

Hopefully not. But interestingly, many people respond to
such advertisements for "clinics" that "specialize" in performing hair transplants.

In the section on quackery, I commented on the dubious
value of any clinic-type operation that promises to restore hair.
But in my opinion, the "clinic" that specializes in performing a
medical procedure such as a hair transplant—and advertises to
promote it—is infringing upon the established code of medical
practice. While the Federal Trade Commission has recently
ruled that physicians may advertise, most medical societies and
their physician-members regard this kind of approach as highly
unethical.

A "clinic" offering hair transplants is usually run by a non-
medical salesman who recruits customers and hires physicians
to perform the procedure for about 20 percent of the surgical
cost. I've never known any physician experienced in cosmetic
surgery who would ever work for this kind of organization.

As with implants, in order to inject a local anesthetic into
the scalp and make the surgical incisions required for a hair
transplant, a medical license is mandatory. Any physician can

be hired to do this, but there's more to performing a transplant than simply removing small sections of scalp. Engaging a hair clinic to overtreat your dandruff will cost you only money, but taking pot-luck on the physician they supply for your hair transplant is chancing something that may damage more than your pocketbook.

Who Should Perform Your Hair Transplant?

Doctors who specialize in hair transplants are usually dermatologists, some are plastic surgeons and a few acquire the training that enables them to perform this procedure.

If you can't find a physician through a personal recommendation from a friend who has had a transplant, you could ask your family doctor, call your local medical society, or write to the American Society for Dermatologic Surgery, Inc., 210 South Grand Avenue, Suite 307, Glendora, California 91740. The members of this surgical society are specialists who have a specific interest in cosmetic surgery.

How to Evaluate the Physician

When you find a physician to consult with, you could, of course, interview *him*.

Inquire about his qualifications. If he calls himself a dermatologist or plastic surgeon, he should have received postmedical school training in a residency program to be *qualified* in his specialty. A qualified specialist can become *certified* in his particular specialty by passing an examination administered by his peers.

Find out if he is a member of your county's medical society. This usually insures that his methods of practicing medicine are consistent with the standards set by your medical community.

Ask about his experience in performing hair transplants.

If you've never met anyone who has had a transplant, ask to see or talk to some of his patients.

Ask about how he performs his hair transplants. Does he do only the minimum surgery legally required and turn most of the procedure over to assistants, or does he do it all himself? The remaining chapters in this section should provide you with a sense of what you should expect from a doctor performing a transplant.

Ask if he will be available to see you the next day, or anytime after your transplanting session, in case a problem arises.

Finally, ask yourself whether or not he's the kind of physician you'd want treating you for other medical problems. A hair transplant, while only a form of minor surgery, is still a medical procedure and should be taken as seriously by you as you would any other kind of medical treatment.

The Physical Qualifications You Require.

After you've convinced yourself that you've found the right doctor, he, in turn, must convince himself—and you—that he has found the right patient.

Being the "right patient" means that you are medically and emotionally suited for a hair transplant.

To satisfy the medical requirements, you should need a transplant, have enough hair to donate for it, and not have any physical disabilities that might interfere with a good result. There are several questions that should be asked by you and your doctor.

Do You Need a Hair Transplant?

The most common "non-candidate" is a person who simply hasn't lost enough hair to warrant a transplant. That person is likely to complain about hairline recession or "thinning."

The recession problem usually occurs in a young man who is upset because he has "lost his hairline." If it appears likely that he may become *very bald* over the years, it is probably unwise to risk restoring his hairline with the limited number of hair grafts that will *eventually remain* . If we satisfy his *immediate* needs, he may wind up with a full hairline and nothing between it and his rear fringe.

Furthermore, if he becomes middle-aged and bald, a recessed transplanted hairline, which may be an anathema to him now, can later become quite desirable. The young man who is just beginning to lose his hair is often the most difficult patient to talk *out* of a transplant.

The other "non-candidate's" problem concerns a man or woman usually in his or her late twenties to early forties, but occasionally younger, who has begun to notice "thinning" over the top of the scalp or crown.

"Thickening" the area might require the removal of balding scalp that still has about half the hair density of the scalp that would replace it. The gain might not be worth the effort. The loss of density must reach the point where a transplant will really make a *significant* difference.

In answer to the commonly asked question, "Shouldn't I start my transplant before my baldness becomes obvious?" I usually answer, "Yes, but you should never sacrifice useful hair as long as careful styling can still work for you."

Do You Have Enough Hair Left to Donate?

The other end of the "non-candidate" spectrum is usually an older person who has lost so much hair that a transplant becomes impractical. Since the transplanted hair is usually donated by the "fringe" at the back of the scalp, that area should not be too thin.

The narrowness of this rear fringe, however, may not be a limiting factor. It is often possible to remove enough hair, if its density is adequate, to create a pleasing cosmetic effect in the frontal area. In general, if the remaining hair is fine, dark in color and sparsely distributed, it may be wise to do nothing.

Who Should Not Risk Having a Hair Transplant?

Anyone whose health is not good should not (and probably would not) undergo any cosmetic procedure.

Anyone having any kind of bleeding tendency would obviously be a poor candidate for any form of surgery.

Anyone who develops abnormal ("keloidal") scarring should avoid all elective skin surgery. A keloid is a scar that grows beyond its original borders. Since keloids are unusual on the scalp, a test graft could be placed and observed for several months.

Anyone who is allergic to local anesthetics should be tested to find one that is acceptable, although the anesthetic we use today has very little allergenic potential.

Emotional Considerations Should Not Be Overlooked

To evaluate a patient's emotional "readiness" for a hair transplant, motivation and attitude are the two factors that seem to count most.

Are You Motivated Properly?

You can't be "talked into" having a hair transplant. Whether you're quite bald or have a limited area that you want filled in, you ·may require several transplanting sessions to achieve the desired effect. Patience is an absolute necessity, because results often accrue slowly.

Do You Have a Realistic Attitude About What You Hope to Accomplish?

People may sometimes expect to be "reborn" by cosmetic surgery. Like most other procedures, a hair transplant will probably not radically change you, nor can it exactly replace what nature has taken away or create what nature has never intended.

When you've found the right doctor, and he's confirmed that you're an acceptable candidate, he should explain how he performs the procedure, what bald area can be treated, how many sessions might be necessary, and how much it will cost.

When all the requirements are satisfied, you're ready to begin.

16

What Common Baldness Is Really About

SEVERAL YEARS AGO, a woman in her early twenties consulted me about having a hair transplant. Because the hair over the top of her scalp had thinned considerably, she qualified for this procedure, which she eventually underwent.

During her initial consultation, she asked the one question that crosses the lips of practically every transplant candidate: "Why am *I* bald?" This problem concerned her, perhaps even more than the average patient, because she was *young, female* and had *no bald relatives*. It seemed to her that she should be the least likely recipient of a condition such as common baldness.

Her case, while slightly atypical, is particularly instructive, because what I told her applies equally to any one of the millions of people past the age of twenty who are bald.

How Our Follicles Fail Us

Many months before we're born, a soft, fine, hairy fuzz begins to grow over our foreheads and scalps. While this velvety cover will persist on our foreheads for a lifetime, our scalps start to nuture hairs that, by birth, will be longer than any other on our bodies.

The major reason our scalp hairs thrive so lavishly is that they're produced by the largest follicles found in our skins. Throughout our early years, these follicles increase in size, shedding their hairs about every two to six years to clear a path for a new hair that grows thicker and longer than the one it replaced. By our late teens our hairs have reached their adult size, populating the scalp in numbers that will never again be equaled.

For most of us entering our twenties, this situation reverses itself because thereafter, we all lose hair. If we're lucky, however, our hair thins gradually and diffusely, so that by our fifties or sixties, we can perceive only a slight decrease in scalp hair density. For the one middle-aged person in four who definitely shows signs of common baldness, he or she will have lost considerable hair in patterns that are quite specific for this condition.

Despite any claims to the contrary, the balding hair follicles are following an inescapable course that was programmed into them during their early development.

For reasons still not understood, most of the follicles residing in the rear and side fringe areas of the scalp continue to produce hair. They seem to be capable of generating enough two-to-six year hair cycles to keep these areas well-covered, if not forever, at least for anyone's average lifespan.

The follicles destined to bald do so gradually. With each new cycle, they become smaller, yielding hairs that grow poorly because they have shortened growth periods and extended resting periods.

By the time these balding follicles enter their final growth cycle, they resemble the follicles that reside in the fetal scalp. After their last cycle, their regression to an earlier life style is complete—they simply disappear.

Common baldness is *not* a disease. It is simply a reversal of a follicle's maturation process back to its earliest form. The scalp of an older bald adult and a very young fetus become similar in one important respect. They both are bald because they both lack hair follicles!

Why Our Follicles Fail Us and What Is Being Done to Correct It

While we now know *how* follicles self-destruct, the accolades eventually will go to the person who can explain *why* it happens and what we can do to prevent it.

We do know that there are three "trigger" factors responsible. Although scientists are carefully studying this problem, the anti-baldness cure is still not quite ready to be delivered to your local pharmacy.

The most undisputed factor is *aging*. Time must eventually claim every scalp follicle, but we're all safe until late adolescence. No matter how barren a scalp may become, *all* its follicles are capable of recycling themselves for enough two-to-six year growth periods to keep our heads well-covered until our teens.

Baldness may begin as early as the late teens or as late as the early sixties. The age at which it starts and the speed at which it progresses relates directly to the number of scalp follicles "programmed" to bald.

By age 25, about 10 percent of American men have recognizable baldness. At age 35, the percentage is about 35 percent; at age 45, about 45 percent; and by age 65, it climbs to 65 percent.

The man blaming his military service for his accelerated hair fall misses the obvious reason. His age—not his drill sergeant—is responsible. The same frequency of balding among his civilian friends in his age group attests to this fact.

Similarly, the unfortunate young woman who consulted me had reached the age when her scalp follicles were programmed to regress. Since common baldness is unusual in young women, she probably had few, if any, acquaintances her age who were experiencing this difficulty.

There is much interest today in uncovering the secrets of the aging process. Since baldness relates somehow to aging hair follicles, hopefully some of this information will be helpful in treating this condition.

Perhaps the answer will come—as often it has in medicine—from some other field that is completely unrelated to the one being studied. Recently a drug, used for treating high blood pressure, was found to encourage growth of body hair. Because one patient seemed to benefit "scalp-wise," the drug is now being investigated for this interesting side effect. It seems to increase certain chemicals in the hair follicle that stimulate its metabolism—that is, it may enable a sluggish follicle to perform better.

The second known factor influencing baldness may prove to be the most challenging to correct. It is *evolution*. This imposing—and usually beneficial—progression of nature has taken us out of the trees, but it has also chosen to disfranchise our scalp hair.

Human evolution has spanned thousands of centuries. During that time, certain traits have spontaneously appeared which, if favorable or simply strong enough, have been passed on to succeeding generations. Baldness is one such strong, albeit undesirable trait. Living in this century, we are under a subtle, but firm, evolutionary pressure to lose body hair, since we no longer require its protection.

The individual losing his or her hair, aware of a lineage of bald ancestors, knows who to blame. On the other hand, someone lacking a family history of baldness, may either have inherited the condition as a "hidden" trait passed on from past relatives or have developed it spontaneously in the way it first occurred in times long past.

The way we inherit our baldness is actually quite complicated and still not well-understood. But if you have many bald relatives, you're certainly more likely to lose your hair. While your mother's family may be slightly more responsible statistically, for all practical purposes, either side will do.

We are now starting to decipher the codes of inheritance. Recently much publicity—and controversy—has been generated by experiments in which inherited traits of simple organisms have been altered in the laboratory. While this type of genetic manipulation is in its infancy, it may someday provide the method for changing the inherited code for baldness that is locked within the hair follicle.

I've already discussed the third baldness "trigger" factor—*male hormone*—in earlier chapters. Without it, a hair follicle, whatever its inherited tendencies or age, is less likely to fail.

Probably this factor will be the first to yield to some type of hair follicle "castration" by a local application of an anti-male hormone substance. Unfortunately, this kind of approach promises to be more useful in slowing down the balding process rather than regrowing hair that has already been lost.

The Classification of Common Baldness

When your follicles finally fail you and you begin to lose your hair, your baldness will usually fit one of several patterns.

I've classified these patterns into four major groups and four less common variations (figures 8, 9). Since baldness is a progressive condition, you may find that at any given time, your pattern only approximates one pattern or shares features of several.

Visualizing the way baldness progresses from minimal to extreme hair loss, may enable you to estimate the future course of your own condition. For example, a forty year old, who has only experienced the minimal amount of hair loss characteristic of a Group 1 pattern, is certainly less likely to reach the extreme baldness of Group 4, than someone half his age who is similarly affected.

Furthermore, the physician and the transplant candidate can use these illustrations to more intelligently plan the placement of hair grafts.

Group 1 baldness exists when the hairline recession produces a definite indentation, or the crown thins, or both occur together.

Group 2 changes occur when the hairline completely inverts and the "bald spot" enlarges. A narrow "bridge of hair" remains to separate these two areas.

Group 3 people lose this "bridge of hair." Their scalps become quite barren, but the rear "fringe" remains—usually quite high—so when viewed from the rear, the hair appears full.

Group 4 constitutes the most advanced stage of hair loss. The rear fringe narrows to take on a "horseshoe" appearance. The remaining hair, residing over the ears and dipping down at the rear, may remain full or become quite sparse.

Variation F (Forelock) is characterized by a forelock or tuft of hair remaining in the center of the hairline. The rear fringe usually retains the height and fullness of Group 3.

Variation T (Thinning) describes a kind of common baldness in which a cover of sparse hair remains over the top of the head. The fullness of this hairy cover usually relates to that of the rear fringe—if dense, the fringe resembles the kind found in Group 3; if sparse, the narrow Group 4 "horseshoe" is more likely.

Variation S (Sides) is fairly uncommon, occurring in less than three per cent of pattern baldness. The only significant loss of scalp hair occurs over the ears on both sides of the scalp.

Variation W (Woman) represents the usual kind of female pattern baldness. Women rarely lose their hair in a way compat-

Figure 8. Four Major Groups of Common Baldness

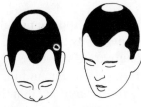

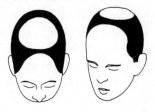

GROUP 1. Frontal recession and/or balding of crown

GROUP 2. "Bridge of hair" remains to separate the bald frontal and crown areas.

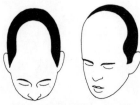

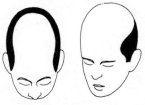

GROUP 3. Baldness from frontal to crown area. Rear fringe remains quite high, reaching crown.

GROUP 4. Rear fringe narrows to "horseshoe" shape.

Figure 9. Four Variations of Common Baldness

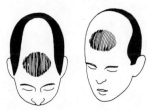

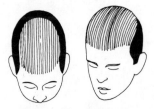

VARIATION F *(Forelock).* Baldness similar to Group 3, but forelock (frontal tuft) remains.

VARIATION T *(Thinning).* Baldness similar to Groups 3 or 4, but sparse hair covers the bald scalp.

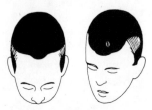

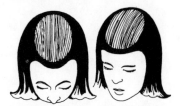

VARIATION S *(Sides).* Hair loss only over the sides of the scalp.

VARIATION W *(Woman).* "Female Pattern" baldness. Narrow rim of hairline remains, but hair thins over the top of the scalp.

ible with the above groups. Similarly, balding men do not often fit into this category.

The hairline retains its rounded "female" appearance along with most of its hair within a ¼ to ½ inch of its border. Behind the hairline, thinning advances enough to permit the scalp to show through. The sides and rear fringe often remain full, but in advanced cases, thinning may become obvious even in these areas.

17

How Hair Is Transplanted

THE BALDEST SCALP contains thousands of transplantable hair follicles, located only inches from where they're most needed. To move them this short distance, three surgical methods have been developed, employing scalp grafts known variously as "flaps," "strips," and "plugs."

While all three methods are used today, most hair transplants are performed with "plug" grafts, because they're simpler and safer to work with and yield the most satisfying results.

The transplant candidate need only be bald enough to justify undergoing the procedure and be endowed with enough side and rear "fringe" scalp hair to make it all worthwhile.

"Flaps"

To create a "flap" or "full thickness" graft, a surgeon cuts out three sides of a rectangular patch of scalp from above the ears and swings it over to the bald area to create a new hairline (Figure 10).

This is a major, in-hospital procedure requiring a great deal of surgical expertise. Although a fairly large portion of bald scalp can be provided with "instant" hair density, this method is fraught with certain problems that detract from its usefulness.

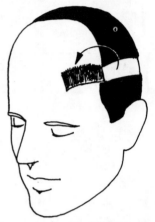

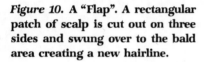

Figure 10. A "Flap". A rectangular patch of scalp is cut out on three sides and swung over to the bald area creating a new hairline.

To insure a proper "take," or graft survival, the blood vessels feeding the transplant must remain intact while they're moved along with it. Because these vessels are quite fragile, they're frequently damaged, resulting in poor graft survival and catastrophic hair loss.

To alleviate this problem, a variation of this type of transplant, known as a "free flap" procedure, has been developed by a team of Japanese surgeons. The "free flap" is cut out on all four sides, completely severing its blood supply. After setting the graft into its new location, the surgeons meticulously reestablish its blood supply to the recipient blood vessels by a delicate microsurgical technique.

But even if this technical obstacle is surmounted, two esthetic problems remain.

The first problem involves the surgical scar that delineates the border between the forehead and transplanted hairline. Little can be done to minimize this scar, except to hide it with bangs or a Caesar-type hairstyle.

The other problem concerns the unnatural direction in which the newly transplanted hair grows. A flap graft cannot provide hair that will grow in the direction of the hair that has been lost. Hairs growing from the sides of the scalp exit much closer to the surface than in other areas. When transplanted to the frontal area, these hairs lie much too flat against the scalp rather than "standing up" in the way they should.

While a "flap" graft may provide a faster way to achieve a high density transplant, the problems of graft survival and poor esthetic results have limited its usefulness.

"Strips"

A surgical "strip" graft is a narrow rectangular patch of scalp, cut out on all four sides, that is usually transplanted to create a hairline (Figure 11).

Unlike the larger "flap," its blood supply needn't be moved along with it or be laboriously reestablished by a difficult microsurgical technique. After being placed into its new location, the adjacent bald scalp sends new blood vessels directly into it.

Like a "flap" graft, however, it must be sewn into place. If it's used to create a hairline, an unsightly scar will again mark its border with the forehead.

While this procedure can be performed in the office rather than a hospital, extreme care must be taken to avoid damaging

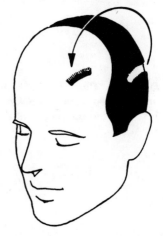

Figure 11. A "Strip". A narrow rectangular patch of scalp is removed from the back of the scalp to create a new hairline.

this delicate graft. Despite the most painstaking precautions, poor "takes" result quite often. "Skip" areas of non-growth are common, and not infrequently the entire graft winds up almost completely devoid of hair.

"Plugs"

When we talk about a "hair transplant," we are usually referring to that procedure in which a small cylinder of hair-bearing scalp—or "plug"—is taken from the rear or side fringe areas and transferred to either the bald crown or frontal region (Figure 12).

While this transplant method requires several sessions to approach the density of hair acquired with a "flap" graft, the ease with which it can be performed, coupled with its superior esthetic results, make it the logical choice for surgically replacing hair.

The hair transplanting surgeon uses a trephine or "punch" to remove the cylindrical section of scalp, properly called a *donor graft* rather than "plug." The graft is quite small, measuring about ⁵/₁₆ inch deep by ³/₁₆ inch diameter.

Figure 13 illustrates a cut-away section of a typical donor

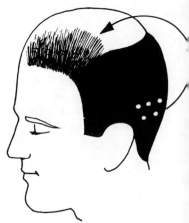

Figure 12. "Plugs": Small cylinders are removed from the back and are inserted into the bald scalp.

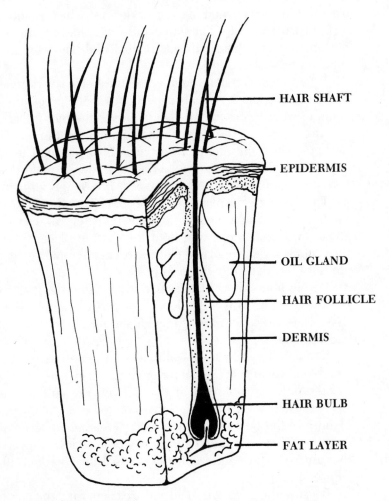

HAIR SHAFT

EPIDERMIS

OIL GLAND

HAIR FOLLICLE

DERMIS

HAIR BULB

FAT LAYER

Figure 13. **Cut-away Section of a Donor Scalp Graft**

scalp graft. The hair follicle is intimately related to all three skin layers. The bulb—or hair-producing portion of the follicle— lies within and is cushioned by the fat, or adipose, layer. The entire follicle is supported by and receives its nourishment from the fibrous portion of skin, or dermis, which is about ¼ inch thick in the scalp. The skin mantle, or epidermis, provides the opening, or "pore", through which the hair exits to the surface of the scalp.

When a donor graft is removed, all three skin layers must be included. The hair is actually superfluous to the procedure—it could even be plucked. All that counts is the hair follicle.

After removing the hair-bearing donor grafts, the physician next "punches" out identical sections of bald scalp. The term "plug" actually refers to the hairless cylinder of scalp that is taken from a bald area. After removal, it is simply discarded.

The donor graft is placed into the void left by the removal of the bald plug. Light pressure is applied for several seconds to allow the blood to clot and hold the graft in place. Because these grafts are so small and clotting occurs so rapidly, stitches are not required to fix them in place.

Within hours, new blood vessels move into the graft from the surrounding skin to feed the new arrival. Within several days, as healing continues, the graft and its adjacent host skin become one.

Keeping the grafts small facilitates easy penetration of these vital blood vessels. When larger grafts, or strips, are used, the blood supply may not reach all the hair follicles—and they die.

Because of their small size, the rounded edges of the grafts blend into the host skin quite evenly, creating an acceptable hairline. While they might appear obvious on close inspection, they are always less noticeable than the scarified borders left by flaps and strips.

Because the grafts are small and are taken from the rear half of the scalp, where the hairs grow "out" in the same manner as the front and crown hairs, they can be directed to exactly duplicate the original pattern of growth in the bald host areas.

Finally, the plug- or punch-graft method is a minor office procedure that, in the hands of an experienced physician, is completely safe, with little to no discomfort for the patient.

18

Why a Hair Transplant Works

IT MIGHT BE QUITE difficult to convince someone who has never seen an airplane that such a heavier-than-air machine could indeed fly.

Similarly, people who have never seen transplanted hair growing often harbor reservations about the validity of this process. The publicity generated by the successful transplantation of other organs, notably hearts, has eased most of these doubts, but nonetheless, nearly everyone questions certain aspects about the way in which a hair transplant works.

Can You Transplant Individual Hairs?

I've heard about schemes that involve implantation of individual hairs—either real or synthetic—into a bald scalp. But they can't work, because a hair without its follicle is simply a foreign body that would be rejected by our skin no matter how it was implanted.

The one thing this procedure isn't is a *hair* transplant—it is a *scalp* transplant, and it's the follicle that really counts. Since the hair follicle is intimately associated with the scalp from which it originated, complete sections of scalp must be transplanted.

While it should, theoretically, be possible to transplant a

thin sliver of scalp containing only a single follicle, a successful "take" usually requires that the donor graft is at least several millimeters in diameter, containing about a dozen follicles. Grafts that are too small—or too large—just do not survive properly.

Will a Bald Scalp Always Accept a Transplant?

The host scalp must only contain a sufficient blood supply in order to feed its donor grafts. The baldest scalp often appears thin and pale, but it usually contains more than enough blood vessels to support a transplant.

Scalps affected by the dandruff-producing conditions, including psoriasis, usually accept transplanted grafts without difficulty. It is advisable, however, to treat the scaling before and after the transplant session to reduce the chances of infection.

Even if a scalp has been scarred by injuries such as burns or radiation or by surgery, the process may still work. As long as the scarring isn't too deep, enough blood vessels usually remain to insure a proper "take."

Will the Transplanted Graft Continue to Produce the Same Type of Hair?

It always does, because a hair transplant is guided by a concept known as "donor dominance." The donor graft, as long as it is placed in a healthy environment, will retain its identity and continue to reproduce its own type of hair. These grafts will continue to grow hair in any area of skin possessing a good blood supply, even if they're relocated to the sole of the foot.

While bald scalp is the usual host area, these grafts have been used to replace lost eyebrows—but the hair still grows as scalp hair, requiring frequent trimming to keep it presentable.

Can You Transplant Hair From Other Parts of the Body to the Scalp?

Since skin is completely compatible with itself, just as a scalp graft will thrive in any other surface area, so will other skin survive there.

The quips made about chest and pubic hair transplants are not unsound—technically. Esthetically, however, the thought of having chest or pubic hair growing atop one's scalp seems somewhat less than appealing.

Does the Transplanted Hair Really Continue to Grow or Does It Fall Out After Several Years?

Many transplant candidates have told me that they'd be satisfied to keep their new hair for about five to ten years. Their expectations, however, should be for a lifetime.

As long as the grafts are removed from the rear fringe of scalp hair, they should continue to recycle themselves almost indefinitely, because that is their "programmed" destiny. Because it is likely that a small percentage of this fringe hair will be shed by the seventh or eighth decade of life, you should expect to lose only that small amount of transplanted hair.

A graft removed from above the rear fringe in an area of scalp that is destined to bald will continue to grow hair in its new location until the day that its ex-neighboring follicles bald. It never forgets its origins.

Can You Take the Hair From Someone Else?

Many of my bald patients have assured me that they have several willing friends or relatives who would be only too happy to donate some of their precious locks for a transplant. While I don't doubt the sincerity of these proposals, the feasibility of such a transfer is, unfortunately, still unrealistic.

Like the implantation of an isolated hair, any attempt to transplant an organ from another individual would result in its rejection by the host. In the case of a heart transplant, the host must be treated with powerful medications that suppress his rejection mechanisms.

This kind of heroic therapy is warranted only for a transplant that is life-sustaining, because it suppresses *all* its host's defense mechanisms. While on such medication, a patient with a simple cold may find it turns into pneumonia. A heart transplant patient is more likely to succumb to the side effects of these suppressive drugs rather than a mechanical failure of his new heart.

Any tissue or organ transplanted from one person to another is known as a *homograft* (homo = human). If the donor graft is taken from the same individual and merely moved to another location, it is called an *autograft* (auto = self). For now, hair transplants work only if they are autografts.

The only exception to this rule involves transplants between identical twins. Since, chemically, they are really the same person, grafts of any kind could be exchanged between them. Unfortunately, if a hair transplant were being considered, choosing the donor would be difficult, since each twin would be affected by the same degree of baldness.

Perhaps future research will provide a method of "desensitizing" homografts. Hair-bearing grafts from willing donors could then be made available to return the baldest scalp back to its juvenile density. Only at that time will you be able to find out how sincere your friends and relatives really are about relinquishing their hair!

19

The Transplant Session

I REMEMBER VIEWING a hair transplant on a television news program in which the commentator warned, "If you have a sensitive stomach, don't watch this!" This kind of presentation has unfairly maligned transplants. In the wrong frame of mind, anything—even childbirth—may be viewed in a highly negative fashion.

A hair transplant is only minor surgery. Unfortunately, people, who are not familiar with this procedure often imagine it to be more complex than it actually is. If you feel apprehensive about having a hair transplant because you've heard "it's bloody," "horrible to watch," etc., you needn't worry. When the procedure is performed carefully, a patient's involvement will be quite limited. The patient whose transplant you'll now view never really "saw" any of it until he approved the photographs for publication.

The typical session that follows was performed on a man in his late twenties who had a receded hairline (Group 1 baldness). During this session, forty grafts were transplanted to the left side of his bald area. Approximately eighty more grafts will be required to return enough hair to this area in order to create a "natural" appearance.

Several weeks before the session, he received his pre-operative instructions.

He was advised to forego a haircut so that his hair would remain long enough to cover and hide the donor and host sites. I'm fond of barbers—but too often, they cut hair too short, creating a "coverage" problem especially on the rear donor area of the scalp.

He was asked to shampoo his scalp the night or morning before the session because he probably would not shampoo again for two days.

He was told to avoid taking aspirins for two weeks prior to surgery because they occasionally slow the clotting capacity of blood.

I suggested that he eat a light meal before the session. Fasting, because it lowers blood sugar, is the most common reason people occasionally become queasy during the procedure.

Finally, he was advised to arrange to stay at home and relax the evening of his transplant. The following day, he would be able to resume his normal activities with very few restrictions.

When the patient arrived at my office, I briefly reviewed the transplanting schedule we had agreed upon at the time of his initial consultation.

He was seated while the nurse trimmed the one-by-three inch rectangular area of hair required for his forty donor grafts (Figure 14).

The next step—injecting the local anesthetic required to deaden the skin—is responsible for the most oft-quoted statement made about a hair transplant: "I've heard that it's painful." It simply is not so.

If a local anesthetic is injected *slowly*, there is little or no pain. To allay the *anxiety* that some people have concerning "needles," I use nitrous oxide (laughing gas, sweet air) as an *optional* pre-anesthetic agent. Dentists use it routinely, especially for children. Used as an *analgesic* (pain-remover), it does

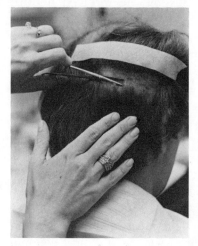

Figure 14.

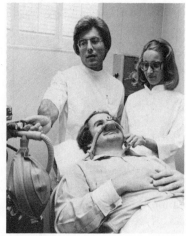

Figure 15.

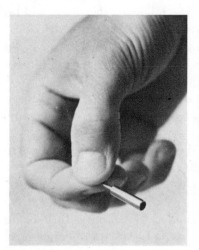

Figure 16.

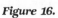

Figure 17.

not put you to sleep, is extremely safe and is quite pleasurable.

This patient breathed the nitrous oxide (Figure 15) for about ten minutes while his donor and recipient areas were injected. Within one to two minutes after discontinuing the gas, its effects completely disappear while the injected areas of scalp remain numb for several hours.

The trephine or "punch" developed for hair transplants is illustrated in Figure 16. It fits into a high speed drill which many of us now use instead of a hand-rotated instrument. This new device permits us to remove better quality grafts than were obtained with the older manual punches.

The patient turned on his side while the donor grafts were removed (Figure 17). He then reclined on his back while the bald "plugs" were incised in the host area. They would be removed later when the grafts were cleansed and ready to be transplanted.

About half the transplanting physicians perform this procedure while their patients are seated rather than lying down. Both "positioning methods" have their proponents, but either seems to work satisfactorily.

About forty-five minutes had passed from the time his hair was trimmed until the grafts were removed. By then, most of the "surgery" was completed. He relaxed for about a half hour while his grafts were cleansed and trimmed.

Preparing the grafts (Figure 18) is the most painstaking part of the procedure. They must be cleansed by passing them through several washes of saline solution (a sterile salt solution that is compatible with all body fluids). Any loose hairs or hairs protruding from the sides of the grafts must be removed to prevent them from acting like irritants which could retard healing.

About half the donor grafts lying in saline solution are illustrated in Figure 19. The grafts are "graded" by the number of hairs they contain. The hairier ones will be placed where they're needed most—in this patient, along his hairline.

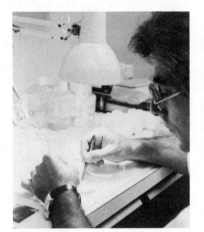

Figure 18.

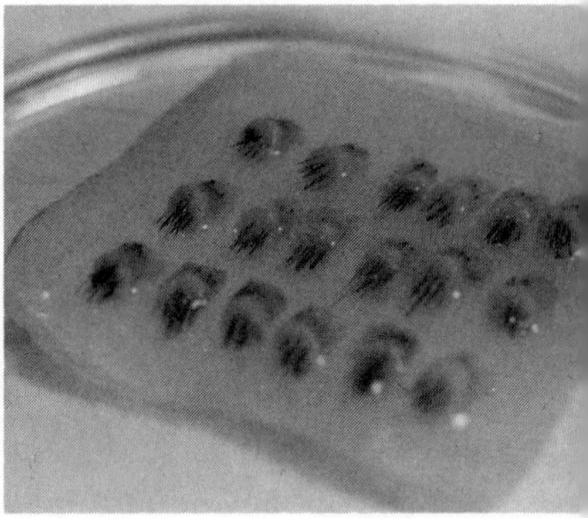

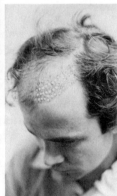

Figure 19.

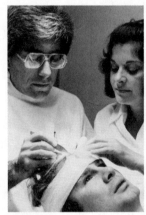

Figure 20.

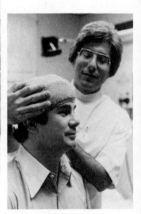

Figure 21.

Figure 22.

Grafts should contain, *on the average*, about twelve or fifteen hairs. Approximately ninety to ninety-five percent of the transplanted hairs should grow. If a graft in a key position does not yield enough hair, part or all of it can be replaced during a later session. The results cannot always be judged on the number of hairs growing from individual grafts. As you'll see later, the final cosmetic effect depends upon the number of grafts and the quality of the hairs that are transplanted.

After the grafts were cleansed and graded, the patient lay down again for about fifteen minutes while the bald "plugs" were removed and the donor grafts inserted in their places (Figure 20). To fix each graft, slight pressure is applied. By the time its neighbor has been inserted, it is firmly in place.

Figure 21 shows the completed transplant. Each graft has been turned so that its hairs exit at a slight angle, facing forward exactly as the lost hair had been directed.

Since about eighty more grafts will be required to create the proper density, spaces have been purposely left between the transplants. Future grafts will fill these spaces to eliminate the tufted "doll-like" effect that may be the hallmark of an incomplete transplant.

When the pressure dressing was applied (Figure 22), about two hours had passed. While the dressing is not absolutely necessary, it can be thought of as a kind of "insurance" to keep the donor grafts in place and prevent bleeding during the night. By the next morning, healing has usually progressed adequately to make bandaging or special care unnecessary.

This transplant, like most, was performed in the office. It is a "clean" surgical procedure requiring sterilization only of instruments and bandages. Gloves and face masks need not be worn.

By the time the patient was ready to leave the office, most of his anesthetic had worn off, but there was no post-operative pain. He drove home by himself, had a comfortable night and returned the next morning to have his bandages removed.

20

When Will the Hair Grow?

A HAIR TRANSPLANT is like sowing seed rather than planting sod, because it takes a while for the new hairs to sprout. There is often confusion about what happens from the time the patient leaves the physician's office until his hair grows. Everyone asks the same questions.

Will I Have Any Pain After the Session?

By the time the head is being bandaged, most of the anesthetic has worn off, and there is no pain. Occasionally, someone will complain of "discomfort" which is easily relieved by an aspirin-type pill. The bulkiness of the bandage may be annoying—"like sleeping with a hat on"—but the first night is usually quite restful.

How Long Is My Head Bandaged?

Overnight. I prefer that patients return to my office the next morning for their dressing removal. It takes about fifteen minutes. Over each graft site—front and back—a crust (scab) forms (Figures 23, 24).

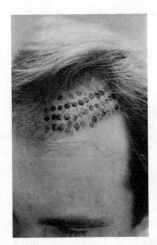

Figure 23.

Figure 24.

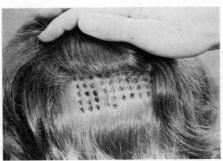

How Long Do the Scabs Stay On?

Anywhere from one to three weeks. The crusts are "natural bandages" that cover and protect the underlying skin. When the scalp is completely healed, they fall off.

Can the Healing Grafts Be Covered?

If you've been "hiding" the bald area with clever styling or a toupee, you would be encouraged to continue doing this until it is no longer necessary. The next day, nobody should know you've had a hair transplant unless you can't—or won't—cover the crusts.

For those people who are unable to hide these crusts and might be embarrassed by them, a hair transplant should either be avoided or undergone during a vacation.

Some individuals are so delighted by the procedure, that the next day they won't hesitate to show their transplants—and scabs—to the world. As you might expect, their enthusiasm is not always shared by those viewing them.

When Can I Resume Normal Activities?

The next day, patients can do anything they like, except engage in stressful exercises. By the end of the first week, there are no restrictions.

When Can I Wash My Hair Again?

With care, you can shampoo the next day. But, if you're hesitant, wait forty-eight hours. If the scalp is shampooed daily, healing will progress rapidly and the crusts will fall off sooner.

What Happens After the Crusts Fall Off?

When the crusts fall off, they usually take the short transplanted hairs with them. Because of the "transplant shock," these hairs stop growing and lose their firm attachment to their follicles. Quite often, when a rounded crust falls off with the short hairs sticking out, it so closely resembles a "shrunken graft" that the patient thinks his transplant "isn't taking." A phone call usually corrects this misinterpretation.

With the crusts gone, each transplanted graft is a circle of bald scalp. Figure 25 illustrates the transplanted area one month after the procedure. Many of the grafts have blended so well into the surrounding scalp, that they can't be noticed.

What Happens to the Donor Area?

The crusts that were covering the donor site will also fall off

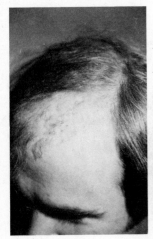

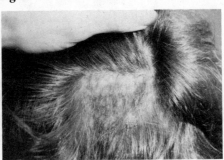

Figure 25.

Figure 26.

within one to three weeks if the area is shampooed daily. During this time, the small holes left by the vacated grafts begin to shrink, forming thin flat scars that are barely noticeable.

Figure 26 shows the donor area one month after the grafts have been removed. The crusts are gone, each donor site is healed and beginning to shrink, and the hair that has been left is getting longer.

Figure 27 shows how well the donor area has healed after six months. Because the holes have shrunk, the hair density appears almost as full as before the transplant. In fact, donor areas may occasionally be "re-used" to provide smaller "fill-in" or "blender" grafts.

Can the Back of Your Scalp Become Bald if Too Many Donor Grafts Are Removed?

Figure 28 shows the rear fringe area of a man *after* 571 donor

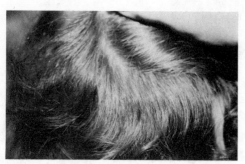

Figure 27.

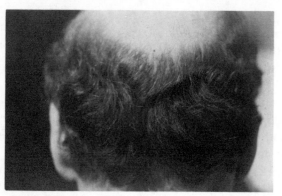

Figure 28.

grafts were removed to fill in the front of his scalp. The fullness
of hair illustrated in the photograph is real. If the donor grafts
are removed with proper spacing, enough hair remains to cover
quite easily.

What Problems May Be Encountered Shortly After a Transplant Session?

In some cases, especially after a hairline has been transplanted, swelling of the forehead may develop within two to three days following the session. It is only a cosmetic inconvenience, because it cannot harm the transplant site. If any swelling does occur, it always disappears within several days.

Post-transplant bleeding practically never occurs if the overnight bandage is applied properly and the patient relaxes the first evening.

Infections develop infrequently, but if they do occur, they are usually limited to only a few grafts, are very superficial and rarely disrupt hair growth.

Occasionally, a donor graft is accidentally pulled out of place within the first few days following the session. If this happens, it's best to forget about it. Over the total number of grafts that are usually transplanted, loss of one—or even several—is meaningless.

What Problems May Persist Beyond the Time of the Transplant?

Numbness in the operated areas—front and rear — may persist for months in some patients. But, with time, it always disappears.

Elevation of the transplanted grafts, or "cobblestoning," occurs occasionally. If it is troublesome cosmetically, the elevations can be flattened by cauterization.

Poor hair growth of several grafts is not unusual. The final results of a transplant, however, should not be judged by the yield of every graft but the total effect. Over the past few years, transplanting techniques have been improved to the point that this distressing problem has been minimized.

Can a Transplant Make the Adjacent Hair Fall Out?

If the hair close to the transplant site is not trimmed before the session, it may be accidentally pulled out. Within a few months, however, this hair will regrow.

If the surrounding hairs are healthy, they should easily withstand the local stresses of the transplant. If this hair seems to thin, most likely it's the result of the progression of the baldness. Sometimes, these surrounding hairs seem to thin out because the stronger transplanted hair contrasts sharply with the poorer quality hair that remains.

When Does the Transplanted Hair Begin to Grow?

Regrowth begins about two and one-half to four months after the transplant. Because the follicles re-establish their cycles independently of each other, the new hairs do not begin to grow at the same time. Figure 29 shows the host area six months post-transplant. Growth started about three months earlier. In this patient, all the frontal hair shown was transplanted.

Does the Transplanted Hair Look Different From the Hair That Once Grew in That Area?

While the hair from the back of the scalp is often wavier, it grows exactly as it had grown before. This hair may, of course, be thicker than the finer hair remaining in the balding area since the stronger, healthier transplanted hair represents the best quality hair the patient possesses.

People occasionally ask if the growing hair "spreads out" like zoysia grass. Unfortunately, in this instance, it grows like sod—strictly from within the confines of the transplanted grafts.

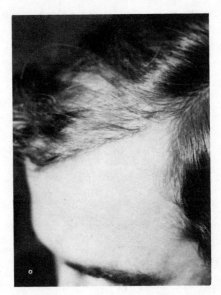

Figure 29.

How Often Can Sessions Be Repeated?

Transplant sessions can be scheduled as frequently as every two weeks, but monthly (or longer) is more advisable since the previous grafts are sure to be healed properly by then.

Can I Have All My Grafts Transplanted in One Session?

The number of grafts transplanted in any one session depends upon two variables.

If the graft *size* is large (within certain limits, the larger the better) and too many are removed from a donor area, they may create a lot of discomfort there, as well as "choke off" the blood supply in the host area, risking graft rejection.

The *area* of the scalp that needs coverage also dictates the number per session. Small areas near the hairline may require the same number of grafts as a larger area further back, simply because the need for density demands more hair. In the patient photographed here, the grafts were purposely spaced one-graft distant from each other so that later grafts could be fit in between the previous ones to provide the closeness that will make for good coverage.

Beware of offers made to transplant an entire head of hair in one or two sessions. This kind of "rapid transplant" is more likely to be offered as a "come-on" by transplant clinics. The hair growth will either be compromised or spaced too far apart to look natural.

When Does the Transplanted Hair Grow Long Enough to Be Cosmetically Useful?

After the three-month "waiting period," the hair that begins to grow lengthens at the same rate common to all scalp hair—about ½ inch a month. Like a pregnancy, about nine months is necessary to develop a useful product.

21

The Numbers

BY THE END OF a consultation, only two questions should remain. The transplant candidate will invariably ask both: "How many grafts will I need?" and "How much will it cost?"

How the Number of Grafts Is Estimated

In general, the more grafts that can be transplanted to any bald area, the better you'll look. The minimum number of grafts, however, that will produce a desirable result depends upon certain variables.

The amount of new hair you require. The balder you are or the more hair density you desire represent the two factors that most directly influence the total number of donor grafts required.

The area of your scalp that must be transplanted. There are only two "critical" areas that require "crowding" of donor grafts—the hairline and the crown. To avoid the "doll-like" effect that is the hallmark of an underdone transplant, many grafts must be placed to re-create either a dense natural hairline or the "whorl" pattern that is characteristic of a crown.

When filling in a bald area between the hairline and crown, fewer grafts are usually needed to achieve a desirable effect, because the spacing will not be obvious to anyone except you or your hair stylist.

The size of donor grafts. The average donor graft diameter ranges between 4 and 4½ millimeters (about ⅜ inch). Smaller grafts are often used as "blenders" to fill in a hairline, and larger grafts may be used if the donor hair density is poor.

I have seen people who have had "bargain" transplants or "fast" transplants of 200 or more grafts per session. In these cases, the donor grafts are invariably smaller, require higher numbers to achieve decent results, and usually yield less hair per graft than larger grafts.

The quality of the donor hair. If the donor hair is curly, fewer grafts may be required to achieve the same effect that can be achieved with straight hair. Conversely, extremely fine hair may demand larger numbers of donor grafts to create enough "body" for a satisfactory result.

The color of the donor hair. Since the highest hair density is found with blonds, less with brunets, and still less with redheads, the number of donor grafts yielding equal numbers of hairs will vary with the hair color.

Aside from these differences in natural hair density, lighter colored hair will cover more effectively, since it contrasts less with a bald scalp.

The healing time of donor grafts. This variable does not actually affect total graft numbers, but it does affect the frequency of transplant sessions. Many people want their hair transplanted as quickly as possible. But, since healing time varies from two to four weeks and the number of grafts transplanted each session varies between forty and eighty, the frequency—and number—of sessions will vary accordingly. Under special circumstances, more grafts can be transplanted more often, but the risks of producing poor hair growth and post-surgical discomfort usually dissuade most people from choosing a "quick" approach.

The numbers of grafts needed for the various stages of common baldness. The following photographs of transplant patients illustrate the typical graft requirements for the four major groups and four variations of common baldness described in chapter 16.

The number of grafts are listed for each patient. The shaded areas in the accompanying line drawings show where the grafts were placed to provide the results seen in the follow-up photographs.

Once you identify your own pattern of baldness, you should gain a sense of how many grafts you'll require for a successful transplant. The variables that were listed above, however, may detract from—or add to—the results achieved in these patients. Aside from these known variables, there are always those unknown factors, common to any medical procedure, that will make these comparisons not quite as exacting as you might hope for.

Group 1 Hairline Recession (Figs. 30 A, B)

To restore his hairline as close to its former state as possible, 133 grafts were transplanted. In this case, the density of the grafts was excellent. Three sessions were required to crowd the grafts close enough to avoid a "doll-like" effect. An equivalent number of grafts were transplanted to the other side of the receded hairline, which is not shown in these photographs.

Group 1 Balding of Crown (Figs. 31 A, B)

To re-create the lost "whorl" pattern, 95 grafts were transplanted. While these grafts have improved his problem, approximately 60 more will be needed to complete the transplant.

Group 1 Advanced Hairline Recession
(Figs. 32 A, B, C, D)

This case illustrates the fact that any classification of baldness cannot be static. This patient's hair loss had advanced to a stage midway between a "late" Group 1 and an "early" Group 3.

It took seven sessions of 355 grafts to fill in the bald frontal area with enough hair to match the density remaining atop the crown. Graft density and placement was good enough to permit this man to comb his hair straight back, exposing his new hairline.

Group 2 "Bridge of Hair" (Figs. 33 A, B, C, D)

The "bridge" was high enough to contribute to the coverage provided by 523 grafts. His part is combed from hair within the "bridge." This is always an advantage, because a part looks better if the remaining hair is used to form it.

Even if his "bridge" recedes in the future, enough coverage has been provided in the frontal area to maintain a good result.

Group 3 Baldness from Frontal Area to Crown, High Rear Fringe (Figs. 34 A, B, C, D)

To fill in these bald areas, 367 grafts were transplanted. This patient still has many good donor sites available that could be used to fill in more of the crown.

Group 3 "Late" (Figs. 35 A, B, C, D)

This man's baldness was actually close to an "early" Group 4.

The photographs do not faithfully reproduce his dark-blond hair color. Typical for blond hair, his donor density was excellent. His side fringe was also high enough to contain his part. Five hundred fifty-four grafts were transplanted to create this full effect which includes a natural hairline.

Group 4 "Horseshoe" Fringe Remaining (Figs. 36 A, B, C, D, 37 A, B, C, D, E)

The first patient (Figure 36) achieved excellent coverage with only 254 grafts because his hair is blond and his graft density was high. The bald scalp above his lost hairline and along his new part was transplanted. In future sessions, more grafts will be placed further back to give more "body" to his hair transplant.

The second patient (Figure 37) displays the same degree of Group 4 baldness as the other man, but his hair is darker and his donor grafts have less density. *All* his available donor grafts, totaling 394, were transplanted to the part side and frontal area of his scalp. While the final result is acceptable, a large bald spot remains (Figure 37E). If a larger area had been transplanted, he would have gained wider but inadequate coverage.

Many people in this Group 4 category are not suitable transplant candidates. If the donor hair is sparse or fine and/or black in color, the potential for adequate coverage may not make the procedure worthwhile.

Variation F Remaining Forelock (Figs. 38, A, B, C, D)

The persistence of a tuft of growing hair on the frontal area of the scalp always enhances the final transplant results.

This man's baldness was actually close to Group 4. Four hundred one grafts were transplanted to a larger area of scalp than it would have been possible to cover if some of these grafts were needed to fill in the front of his hairline. His side fringe was high enough to contain the part and still contribute hair to the transplanted area.

Variation S "Side" Baldness (Figs. 39 A, B)

This uncommon pattern of baldness is usually difficult to transplant, because many grafts may be required unless the area is small.

Because this man's overall hair density was thin, he had difficulty hiding his "side" baldness. After forty grafts were transplanted to each side, the fullness of these areas had increased enough to satisfy him.

Variation T Thinning of Hair Over the Top of the Scalp (Figs. 40 A, B, C, D)

This patient's pattern of baldness really fits into Group 4. It is designated as "Variation T," because sparsely distributed strands of hair remained over the scalp from the hairline to the rear fringe.

All his available donor grafts (611) were transplanted to the frontal area and crown area adjacent to his part.

Because his hair was quite fine, he could not achieve full density, but the final result was satisfactory. His hair, while thinned, does not look "transplanted," and his density is adequate for a man in his early sixties.

Variation W Woman or "Female Pattern" Baldness (Figs. 41 A, B, C, D)

This woman's problem clearly illustrates the female variant of common baldness. Her hairline remained intact, but behind it, her hair had thinned so much that her scalp was visible.

After only two sessions providing 95 grafts, she regained enough density to provide adequate coverage. Although she let her hair grow out to its natural grey color, she actually had enough new hair density to dye her hair and still maintain coverage.

Many women displaying this pattern, unfortunately, possess sparse hair in their rear and side fringe areas. Some women, who are acceptable candidates, may achieve greater density with transplants, but still must lighten and/or curl the hair to hide their scalps adequately.

The Cost of a Transplant

The physician's fee will reflect his experience with this procedure, the extent of his active participation during a session, his follow-up services, his office facilities and the training of his assistants. If you're offered a "bargain," chances are that some of these factors will be compromised.

The fees, usually "by the graft," average between $10 to $20. Aside from the above factors, this variation also reflects the differences in medical overhead costs in different areas of the country.

Common to cosmetic surgical procedures in general, hair transplant payments are usually made on an "as-you-go" basis. Reimbursement from medical insurance plans is practically non-existent. As of 1976, however, you could write off your transplant as a bona fide medical expense (IRS Ruling 76-332). If you must incur travel expenses, you might qualify for additional "per diem" write-off of about $50 a day.

Most physicians charge a fee for a consultation, which usually equals their fee for an initial office visit. If you're asked for a deposit to reserve your transplant time, the physician is probably allocating this time specifically for you and not scheduling other patients during your session.

There is one future cost factor you should not neglect—the money you must spend for the services of a good hair stylist once your transplanted hair starts to grow. I have seen people who, after spending several thousand dollars for a transplant, did not bother to have their new hair cut properly. The difference between only gaining "more hair" rather than enjoying "better hair" is often decided by your barber or beautician.

As with any kind of cosmetic surgery, your eventual satisfaction cannot be guaranteed. But hair transplantation probably has one of the highest "appreciation rates" of any other cosmetic enhancement procedure.

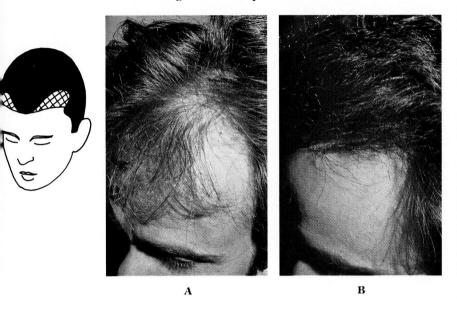

Figure 30. Group 1: Hairline Resession

A B

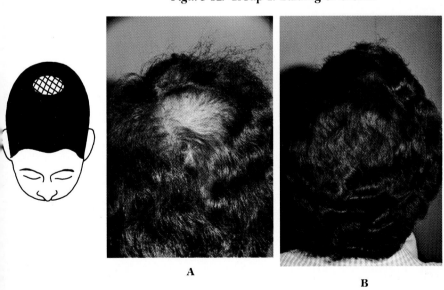

Figure 31. Group 1: Balding of Crown

A B

Figure 32. Group 1: Advanced Hairline Recession

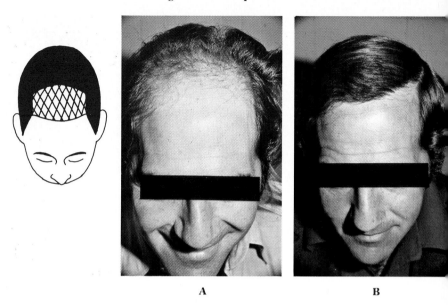

A   B

C   D

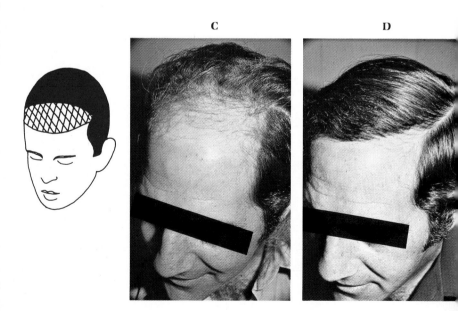

Figure 33. Group 2: "Bridge of Hair"

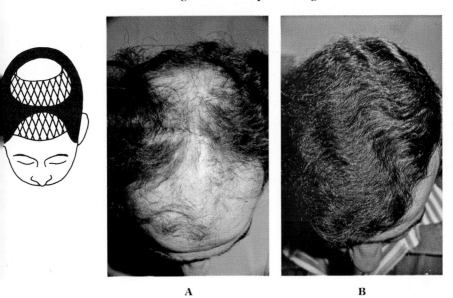

A   B

C   D

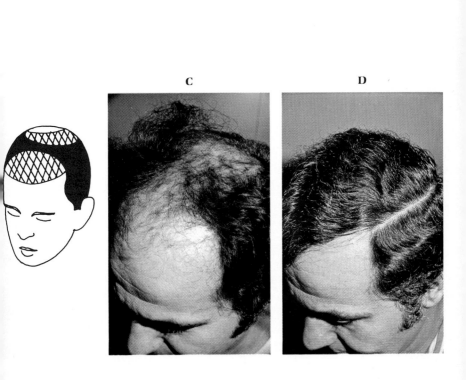

Figure 34. Group 3: Baldness from Frontal Area to Crown.
High Rear Fringe

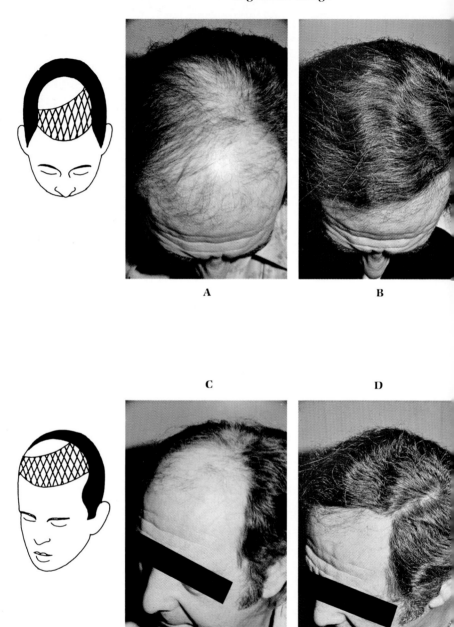

A
B

C
D

Figure 35. Group 3: "Late"

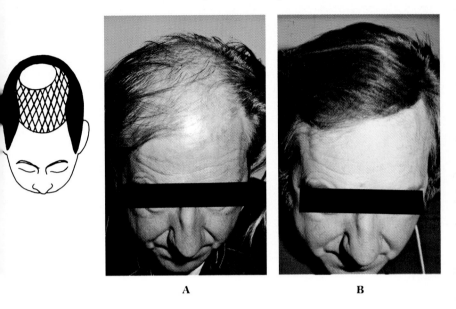

A   B

C   D

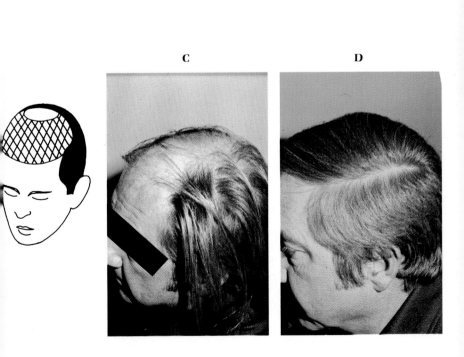

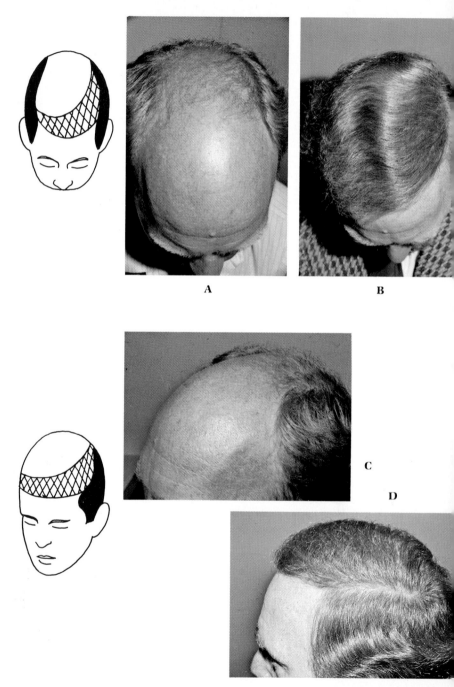

Figure 36. Group 4: "Horseshoe" Fringe Remaining

A

B

C

D

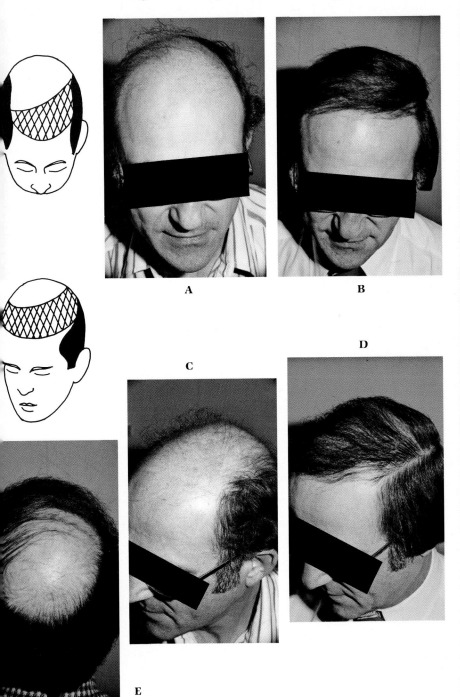

Figure 37. Group 4: "Horseshoe" Fringe Remaining

A

B

C

D

E

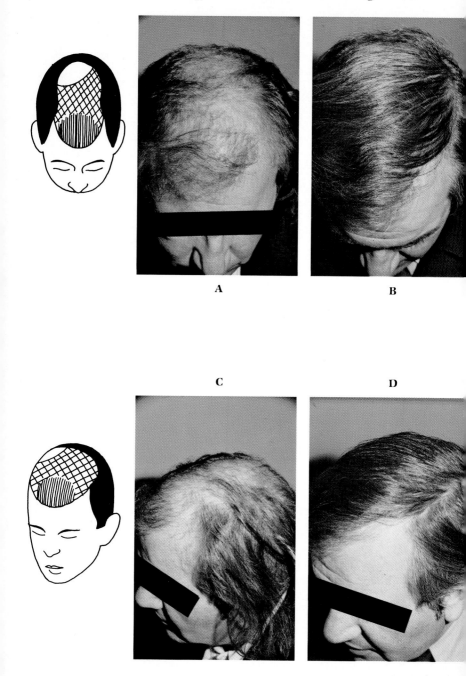

Figure 38. **Variation F: Remaining Forelock**

A

B

C

D

Figure 39. Variation S: "Side" Baldness

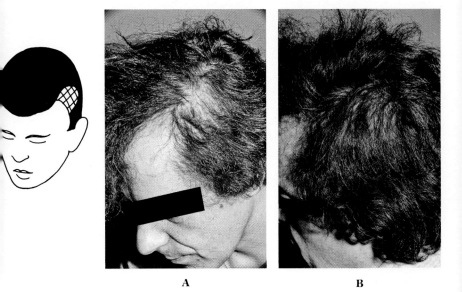

A   B

Figure 40. Variation T: Thinning of Hair Over the Top of the Scalp

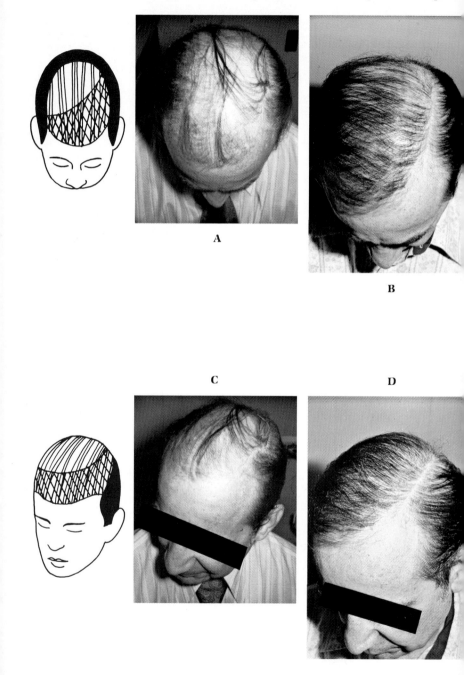

A

B

C

D

Figure 41. Variation W: Woman or "Female Pattern" Baldness

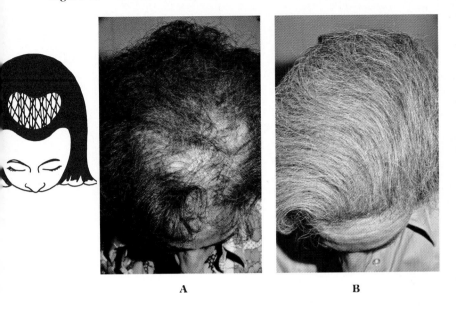

A   B

C   D

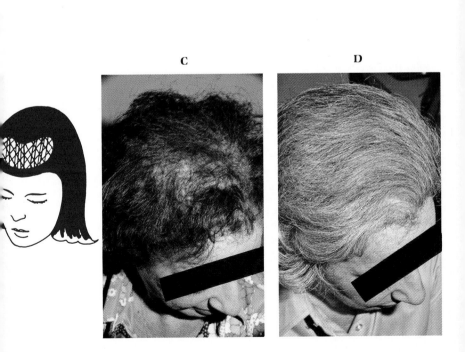

VI

The Unisex Hair Guide

OCCASIONALLY, hair problems display a distinct sexual linkage. But most often, these problems—and their solutions—are distinctly "unisexual."

In the first section of this guide, I've listed various hair types and described the grooming and styling aids available for dealing with them.

My suggestions, however, are not meant to be rigidly applied to every situation. For example, while a short hair style is recommended for fine, straight hair, you may prefer—and look better with—a longer hairstyle. While certain shampoos and conditioners usually work best for certain hair types, the kinds of grooming aids you use may vary with changes in climate and environment, or your work and activities.

In the second section, I've described the ways in which hair sheds and thins so that you can better evaluate your problem—if it exists—and deal with it correctly.

Where indicated, I've listed page references for further explanation in the text. If a sexual linkage predominates, I've noted it in the guide.

22

Grooming and Styling Guide for all Hair Types

Hair Type: Normal

Normal, as opposed to fine or coarse, refers to the size (diameter) of your hair. For discussion of shape (curly or straight), density (thick or thin), or texture (oily or dry) see below.

Shampooing. Shampoo every one to three days. Clean hair has more "body" because it's free of the accumulated oils and dirt that encourage matting.

For suggested products, see p. 67, 68.

Conditioning. Creme rinses (p. 79,80) help control fly-away and restore sheen to hair dulled by some shampoos and hard water.

Instant conditioners (p. 80, 81) benefit hair that has been damaged by sun, heat, chlorinated water, dry winter air, and coloring, perming and straightening agents.

Setting lotion conditioners (p. 82) and hair sprays (p. 83) can be used as desired to set and hold hair in place.

Coloring. Dye or bleach hair as desired (p. 87-92).

Perming or Straightening. Reshape hair as desired (p. 84-87).

Styling. The way in which normal hair is styled depends upon its shape and density. See below and chapter 11.

Hair Type: Fine

Shampooing. Shampoo at least every three days if dry; perhaps daily if oily. Even slight oiliness may mat together fine hair.
For suggested products, see p. 66, 67, 68.

Conditioning. Condition after each shampoo to reduce fly-away and to promote body.
The most useful products include instant conditioners (p. 80, 81), deep-down conditioners (p. 81) and setting lotion conditioners (p. 82). The setting lotions usually come in an "extra body" variety.
Avoid the stiff look of hair sprays, especially the "extra hold" kind.

Coloring. Permanent and semi-permanent dyes will coat and swell the hair shaft increasing its diameter. Henna treatments are often used for this thickening effect (see p. 88).

Perming. The appearance of fullness can be enhanced by a "body wave" (p. 84, 85).
Remember that fine hair requires more cautious use of perming products to avoid hair breakage.

Styling. Fine hair usually looks better (has more body) with a short, blunt cut.

Hair Type: Coarse

Shampooing. Shampoo every one to three days if hair tends to be normal or oily. For suggested products see p. 66, 67.
Shampoo every three to four days if hair tends to be dry. For suggested products, see p. 67, 68.

"Dry hair" shampoos are useful for any kind of coarse hair that is washed often. Coarse hair tends to be dry and difficult to manage even with normal scalp oil production. If you shampoo often and lather only once, enough natural oil should remain to enhance manageability.

Conditioning. To improve manageability, condition after each shampoo with an instant conditioner (p. 80, 81).

Setting lotion conditioners (p. 82) and hair sprays (p. 83) help to control coarse hair.

Coloring. Dye or bleach hair as desired (p. 87-92).

Perming or Straightening. Reshape hair as desired (p. 84-87). Since stronger products may be required to change the shape of coarse hair, you can avoid hair breakage by not attempting to accomplish too much.

Styling. Coarse hair usually looks better with a layered cut worn longer (chapter 11).

Hair Type: Thick

Thick refers to hair density. If you possess a lot of scalp hair, first count your blessings, then refer to this guide for your hair size (normal, fine or coarse), shape (curly or straight), and texture (oily or dry).

Try not to have your hair "thinned out" because this creates shorter hairs of irregular lengths that are difficult to manage.

Hair Type: Thin

Thin means that your hair density is sparse enough to allow your scalp to show.

Shampooing. Shampoo as often as necessary to keep your hair slightly dry. Thin hair that is kept clean and dry will have more body because it is less likely to mat.

Unless your hair is very oily, use shampoos recommended for fine hair (p. 67, 68).

Conditioning. After each shampoo, use an instant conditioner (p. 80, 81) or a deep-down conditioner (p. 81) for their body-building capabilities.

Before styling your hair, use a setting lotion conditioner (p. 82) to further enhance body.

When hair is in place, a light application of hair spray (p. 83) helps to maintain its fullness.

Coloring. Lightening the color of your hair will reduce the contrast between it and your scalp, enhancing the illusion of density.

Permanent and semi-permanent dyes will coat and swell the hair shaft, increasing its diameter. Henna treatments are often used for this thickening effect.

For discussion of bleaching and dyeing hair, see p. 87-92.

Perming. Waving or curling hair usually enhances the illusion of density because each hair covers more scalp. This effect seems to work better with coarse rather than fine hair (p. 84, 85).

Styling. Choose your stylist well.

Keep your hair cut short.

Women often find bangs useful to cover the scalp while some men choose a "Caesar" hair style for the same reason.

Blow-drying your hair should help to promote body.

Partial hairpieces may help (p. 104).

Avoid any heat or massage treatments that promise to thicken hair. They will probably only promote hair breakage.

Avoid damaging your remaining hair by styling methods involving tight rollers, ponytails and teasing.

Hair Type: Curly

Shampooing. For curly hair that is normal, fine or coarse, shampoo as described above.

For fine and/or "frizzy" (tightly curled) hair, frequent shampooing enhances body by eliminating the oiliness that mats hair together.

If you want to temporarily reduce the curliness of your hair, shampoo often and follow the conditioning and styling steps described below.

Conditioning. Condition your hair as directed for size (normal, fine or coarse) and texture (oily or dry), but since curly or frizzy hair worn naturally looks better moderately dry, don't over-condition.

When temporarily relaxing curly or frizzy hair, you'll find setting lotion conditioners (p. 82) are particularly useful.

Coloring. Color hair as desired (p. 87-92), but when using tints or bleaches on hair that has been straightened, make sure to wait at least one week after straightening before coloring to reduce the chance of breakage.

Straightening. Straightening or "relaxing" hair permanently is best done professionally.

If you choose to do it yourself, see p. 86, 87.

Normal to coarse hair tolerates stronger straightening chemicals than fine hair. Larger-diameter hair may accept straighteners every four to six months while finer hair should be left alone for at least nine to twelve months between straightenings.

Frizzy hair is usually impossible to completely uncurl. It can only be partially "relaxed."

Styling. If you choose to wear your hair curly, short, blunt scissor cuts usually work best.

To temporarily relax your curly hair, shampoo, condition, towel dry, apply a setting lotion ("extra hold" if necessary) and blow dry. Follow the same steps for a body wave, but set your hair on large rollers before applying the setting lotion.

Hair Type: Straight

Shampooing. Since straight hair possesses less natural body than curly hair, shampoo as often as possible to keep hair on the dry side to prevent matting (i. e., loss of body).

Select shampoos recommended for normal, fine or coarse hair types.

Conditioning. Condition after each shampoo to enhance body. All types of conditioners are useful (see p. 78-83).

Coloring. Dye or bleach hair as desired (p. 87-92).

Perming. Body waving, aside from improving body, will impart a "softer" look to straight hair (see p. 84, 85).

Coarse hair may require stronger perming solutions. Be careful not to damage hair.

Styling. As a general rule, fine straight hair looks better short, while coarse hair can be worn longer. Women have the option to wear this hair type long and pulled back or up.

Layered hair cuts work well for straight hair (chapter 11).

Hair Type: Oily

Shampooing. Shampoo oily hair often—preferably every day. During the summer or after exercising, if oiliness increases, this hair type may require twice daily shampooing.

The products recommended for oily hair are listed on p. 67.

If the oiliness of your hair is associated with a scaly scalp, try the anti-dandruff products (p. 76, 77). If your oiliness returns several hours after shampooing and is associated with redness and scaliness of your scalp and/or face, you should probably consult with a dermatologist.

Conditioning. Creme rinses (p. 79, 80) usually help oily hair that is difficult to control after shampooing or dry hair that is associated with an oily scalp. All the listed products are essentially "oil free."

Styling. Short hair blown dry usually looks best. Additionally, shorter hair is easier to shampoo frequently.

Hair Type: Dry

Shampooing. Even though your hair and scalp are dry, they still must be cleansed regularly. Try to shampoo at least once or twice weekly. If you use a mild shampoo and lather only once, you should not aggravate your dryness problem.

For suggested products, see p. 67, 68.

Conditioning. Instant conditioners (p. 80, 81) and deep-down conditioners (p. 81) should be used after shampooing.

If your scalp is also dry, try a professional or home "hot oil" treatment as often as necessary (p. 81). You might find it easier to rub olive oil, mineral oil, or a commercial bath oil into your scalp about a half hour before shampooing. These treatments usually provide temporary relief.

Coloring, Perming and Straightening. These procedures (chapter 10) should probably be performed professionally since care must be taken not to further dry the hair and increase its brittleness.

Styling. Brushing with a soft brush may help to distribute your natural oil.

When blow drying, use the lowest setting. Avoid the extreme heat of driers, electric rollers and hot combs.

Avoid excess hair spray as it may promote dullness of the hair cuticle.

Try a cream or oily hair dressing to help lubricate your hair and scalp.

Hair Type: Damaged

Hair may be damaged by "over-processing" (i.e., too much dyeing, bleaching, perming or straightening) and excessive sunlight, heat or back-combing (teasing). All processed hair is slightly compromised and usually requires special handling.

Damaged hair may appear dull, limp, frizzy; it may break easily and have split ends.

Shampooing. Damaged hair must still be cleansed at least once or twice weekly. The proper use of conditioning and baby shampoos should not promote further damage.

For suggested products, see p. 67, 68.

Conditioning. Deep down conditioners (p. 81) used after each shampoo are most helpful.

Coloring, Perming and Straightening. Absolutely *refrain* from any further processing. If your hair is hopelessly damaged, cut it short and buy a wig. When it grows out, you can modify it as desired but with more care.

Styling. Shorter hair styles will probably be easier to manage. Avoid prolonged or excessive heat when blow drying hair. Cut off split ends.

23

Guide for Falling and Thinning Hair

Falling hair is always obvious to the person experiencing it. A physician can verify this complaint by a simple maneuver known as the "pull test." By grasping a group of hairs and *gently* pulling outward, hairs about to be shed are easily removed. Healthy growing hairs cannot be extracted in this way. The force required to remove them must be quite strong (and painful). To "pull-test" your own hair: Shampoo and don't comb or brush for 24 hours. Grasp and gently pull at groups of hairs over your entire scalp. If, during the next 24 hours, you can collect over a hundred hairs, your shedding may well be significant.

Hair thinning may develop gradually over months or years or become obvious within several weeks. Your personal evaluation is most significant. Some people who appear to have normal scalp hair density may actually have experienced a lot of thinning.

The most common types of hair fall and thinning are listed below in order of decreasing frequency. For a full discussion of each type, references to the text are provided.

Gradual Thinning Over Entire Scalp. No Obvious Increase In Daily Hair Fall.

Thinning occurs slowly over months to years. It is usually

noticed in middle age. The "pull test" reveals no increase in daily hair fall. See *Aging*, p. 36.

Gradual Thinning Over Top Of Scalp. No Obvious Increase In Daily Hair Fall.

This is *Common Baldness* (see p. 36, 37). Hairline recession and/or thinning of the crown is usually present. The side and rear fringe remains thick. The "pull test" may occasionally reveal an increase in daily hair fall.

For a discussion of the female variant of common baldness, see p. 130-132, illus. p. 131.

Increased Hair Fall Over Entire Scalp, Little To No Apparent Thinning.

This may normally occur over periods of weeks or months. The "pull test" may reveal a daily increase in hair fall of up to 100-200 hairs.

For a full discussion, see *Daily Hair Fall*, p. 38.

Increased Hair Fall Over Entire Scalp, Thinning Is Quite Obvious.

This usually occurs within several months. The "pull test" usually delivers clumps of hairs with small whitish "roots" (see resting hairs, p. 38) numbering in the hundreds.

The common causes of this massive shedding include *Pregnancy and Birth-Control Pills* (p. 15, 16, 39), *Physical Stress* (p. 39, 40) and The *"Scaly-Scalp" Conditions* (p. 38, 39, 71).

Rapid Hair Fall Creating Single Or Multiple Bald Patches

Alopecia Areata (p. 26, 39) may create bald spots within days or weeks on the scalp or any other hairy area. The "pull test" usually delivers large numbers of hairs around the edges of the bald patches.

Self-induced hair pulling, known medically as trichotillomania (trik"o-til"o-ma'ne-ah), may create thinned patches that look similar to alopecia areata except that broken stubble hairs are found in the patches and the "pull test" is normal. See *Emotional Stress* p. 39.

Rapid Hair Fall Creating Thinning Over The Entire Scalp.

This may occur because of damage to the hair shaft. Over a period of weeks, large numbers of broken hairs may be shed daily. The "pull test" delivers easily-broken "rootless" hairs.

For a full discussion, see Hair Breakage, p. 40.

Index